"OUR GALLANT DOCTOR"

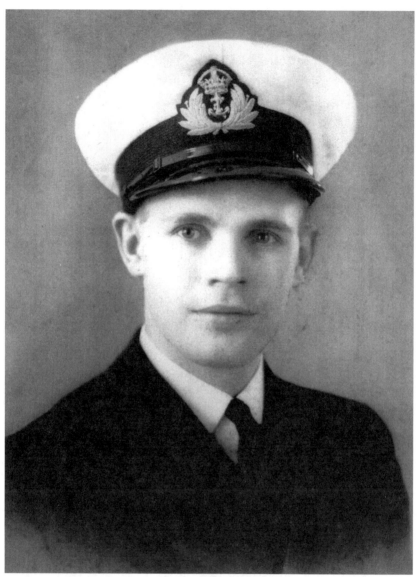

Surgeon Lieutenant George Ainslie Hendry, RCNVR. (Courtesy of Dr. James Goodwin.)

"OUR GALLANT DOCTOR"
Enigma and Tragedy:
Surgeon Lieutenant George Hendry
and HMCS *Ottawa*, 1942

by James Goodwin

with forewords by
Michael Bliss, CM, PhD and
Tony German, Commander RCN (Ret'd)

DUNDURN PRESS
TORONTO

Copy-editor: Jennifer Gallant
Design: Alison Carr
Index: Dennis Mills
Printer: Tri-Graphic Printing Ltd.

Library and Archives Canada Cataloguing in Publication

Goodwin, James
      Our gallant doctor : enigma and tragedy : Surgeon Lieutenant George
Hendry and HMCS Ottawa, 1942 / James Goodwin.

Includes bibliographical references.
ISBN 978-1-55002-687-0

      1. Hendry, George. 2. Ottawa (Ship). 3. World War, 1939-1945--
Campaigns--Atlantic Ocean. 4. Canada. Royal Canadian Navy--
Surgeons--Biography. 5. Ship physicians--Canada--Biography.
I. Title.

D779.C2G65 2007   940.54'5971092   C2007-900083-5

1   2   3   4   5   11   10   09   08   07

Conseil des Arts
du Canada

Canada Council
for the Arts

Canada

ONTARIO ARTS COUNCIL
CONSEIL DES ARTS DE L'ONTARIO

We acknowledge the support of the Canada Council for the Arts and the Ontario Arts Council for our publishing program. We also acknowledge the financial support of the Government of Canada through the Book Publishing Industry Development Program and The Association for the Export of Canadian Books, and the Government of Ontario through the Ontario Book Publishers Tax Credit program, and the Ontario Media Development Corporation.

Printed and bound in Canada.
Printed on recycled paper.

www.dundurn.com

Dundurn Press	Gazelle Book Services Limited	Dundurn Press
3 Church Street, Suite 500	White Cross Mills	2250 Military Road
Toronto, Ontario, Canada	High Town, Lancaster, England	Tonawanda, NY
M5E 1M2	LA1 4XS	U.S.A. 14150

In loving memory of

Betty Summers
(Elizabeth Audrie Minogue)
1918–2006

and

Latham Brereton "Yogi" Jenson
1921–2004

"Show me a hero and I will write you a tragedy."

— F. Scott Fitzgerald

Table of Contents

Foreword:

Fathers and Sons: The Lost Age of Medical Heroism

The history book you are about to read is a breathtaking, classic story of personal, military, and medical heroism. My dear friend and my late brother's dear friend and classmate in medicine, Dr. James Goodwin, presents in these pages a world we have largely lost — a world of courage, duty, sacrifice, and enormous strength of character demonstrated by weak and ordinary young men.

This is intense drama. If it is ever translated to film it will be almost unbearably vivid — a true wartime tale of human frailty, lost love, almost unbelievable surgical daring and stoicism, overwhelming random violence, ghastly death, the final silence of the oil-smoothed sea, and the loneliness of lost lovers who live on almost to our times.

It is a magnificent war story, one of the most remarkable we have from the great days of Canada's contribution to the Second World War. It is a hugely sad personal tragedy, the story of a young man entrapped by a single night of passion into a loveless marriage, from which the only escape seems to be service and sacrifice. But it is also a story of medicine and its values in an age that only a shrinking few of us still remember — the age before miracle treatments, high technology, insurance, bureaucracy, and shifting social values changed forever the meaning of being a doctor.

Medicine used to be a much more personally challenging profession than it is now. It was not hard to be admitted to studies in medicine, partly because the risks of being a doctor were very considerable and the rewards of the career were not always tangible. Risks? Notice that the hero of this book, George Hendry, is the second in his family to die while practising his profession: in 1933 his brilliant brother, Jack, gold medallist in his class, a splendid medical career opening up before him, is bitten by a laboratory monkey and dies of respiratory paralysis. Before the age of antibiotics and other miracle therapies, you often took your life in your hands to practise surgery and medicine. Perhaps more to the point — and this is still the existential barrier that confronts every medical student in our time — the doctor held other people's lives in his hands. It was god-like power, responsibility and challenge, given to humans with anything but god-like abilities, and it could be terrifying almost beyond belief.

It could also be exhausting. Those stories we all remember of heroic country doctors, struggling for hours to reach sick patients — perhaps operating for hours on kitchen tables by lantern light — are prototypes of the surgical climax of this book, as George Hendry tries to save patients' lives in a pitching, tossing, gerry-made operating room in the middle of the North Atlantic, with Nazi submarines literally lurking in the shadows. He probably felt by then that he was a lost soul, but he persevered. I have a vivid memory of coming down to breakfast one morning at about age thirteen and seeing my father, an ordinary country physician, sitting ashen-white at the breakfast table after a night spent in a futile attempt to save a mother and child. In another two years my father would be dead of overwork.

As Goodwin points out in lovely passages in Chapter Two, that generation of medical teachers and students, often literally medical fathers and sons, was often stronger in its idealism and dedication than in its professional proficiency. These kids and the crusty eccentrics who taught them were trying to do a little bit of good for humanity, trying to live out what Osler and the other patron saints of medicine saw as a secular vocation. When things went right, the satisfactions of the medical career must have been intense; as often as not the strains of personal living could undercut and ruin everything.

Jim Goodwin brings to this story not only his considerable passion and perfectionism as an amateur historian (I have always thought the amateur historians, like amateur athletes, are the best and purest of us all) but his own intimate experience with the medical world he describes. His father knew the Hendrys, he knew the Hendrys, he knew University of Toronto medicine just as the classic age was drifting to conclusion in the fifties, he knew what it meant to be a son challenged to live up to his father's expectations. I have always believed that one way to understand Ernest Hemingway's lifelong search for the roots of courage is to see him as a doctor's son.

It goes without saying that Dr. Goodwin is still a book or two shy of having achieved Hemingway's literary stature. But if you read this story carefully and think about it, you will come to realize that it has layers and layers of meaning. For the young it is about a world gone by, including a medical world now about to disappear. For a few of us, the intermediate generation, the sons of the fathers, whether medical or military, it is a book about the values passed on to us by heroic, tragic figures to whom we owe incalculable debts.

Michael Bliss, CM, PhD
University Professor Emeritus,
University of Toronto

Foreword:
Dr. Hendry and HMCS *Ottawa*

*O*ur *Gallant Doctor* is a richly illustrated and quite unusual addition to the field of Canadian naval historiography. Its climax is the loss of HMCS *Ottawa*, torpedoed twice by a U-boat and sunk in mid Atlantic near midnight on September 13–14, 1942, with most of her crew while escorting westbound Convoy ON 127. Had she been equipped with 271 surface warning radar — as were all escort ships of the RN by this time — rather than the Canadian navy's inferior and outdated 286M — she could well have survived and, quite possibly, sunk her enemy. Indeed, 114 very brave men might have been spared.

The author, James Goodwin, has given us an especially intriguing picture of a Canadian wartime ship's company. Individuals' stories and perceptions abound. Among them are the First Lieutenant, Tom Pullen, and Sub-Lieutenant "Yogi" Jenson — the gunnery officer and outstanding author/artist whose drawings illuminate and enrich the book. These two, in particular, provided the author with closely observed and perceptive background on Lieutenant Commander Larry Rutherford, the commanding officer who was lost with his ship, the "gallant doctor" of the title, and many from the lower deck. Particularly ironic is Jenson's account of a 271 radar set being delivered to the ship in Londonderry before she sailed to escort ON 127. He reported this to the captain, who replied that Naval Service Headquarters had dictated that 271 was *not* to be fitted to RCN destroyers as its antenna assembly would have to replace the main gunnery armament's rangefinder/director.

Most unusual in non-fiction of this nature, the book has a well-developed central character — the ship's medical officer, Surgeon Lieutenant George Hendry, RCNVR. He had joined the wartime navy to escape a misguided, disastrous marriage, gained respect and friendships in *Ottawa*, and developed close relationships with the lower deck. Then, during the stormy passage leading to her loss, he performed two emergency abdominal surgeries — one on a sailor with acute appendicitis, the other on a badly wounded DEMS gunner from a torpedoed merchant ship. His "scrub nurse" on both occasions was Tom Pullen. Sadly, both patients died. So, after *Ottawa* went down, did George Hendry. *Our Gallant Doctor* is a fitting memorial to him and to HMCS *Ottawa*.

Tony German, Commander RCN (Ret'd)
Author of *The Sea is at Our Gates: The History of the Canadian Navy*

Preface

$\mathcal{I}$ didn't realize that this was a story that needed telling until many years after George Hendry's death in the war. We Goodwins had a very close family link with the Hendrys. My dad, James C. "Jimmie" Goodwin, was first an assistant to George's father, Professor W.B. Hendry, then a colleague and a close friend. Soon after his father, the much beloved "Chief," died in March 1939 and after he had finished his postgraduate training, George joined my father in practice and took up a junior teaching appointment in the university's department of obstetrics and gynaecology. Though I was but ten years old at the time, I clearly remember George giving my younger brother John and me hockey gloves at Christmas in 1940. I was always a bit of a nerd and my much more athletic brother made far better use of this gift than I did!

When George Hendry was lost in 1942, my dear mother, with a typically maternal penchant for exaggeration, invented a fanciful account of how George, being the great university athlete that he was, swam into the sinking *Ottawa* three times attempting to rescue shipmates and only managed to swim out twice. His framed photograph in naval uniform (the frontispiece and cover for this book) stood on a table in our north Toronto living room for several years after his death. George's mother — all her men gone — lived alone with her memories in an upper duplex on North Avenue Road in Toronto. For several years, I used to take presents and flowers up to her door at Christmas and on anniversaries. It was all very sad.

This was the sum of all I knew about George Hendry's heroism and death until the week after my father's sudden death in August 1953. Wing Commander Hugh Bright, the commanding officer of the Institute of Aviation Medicine, then made his stunning revelation of George's abrupt exit from Toronto and his entry into the navy. I was grieving for my father and I was in the middle of my professional education as a doctor, so I suppose that the thought that this had the potential of a strong story did not cross my mind. I finished medical school, did internship and postgraduate training in Toronto and Boston, then carried on with a research fellowship in Oxford and finally took up several academic teaching/clinical/research posts in Edmonton, Toronto, St. John's, and overseas in Iran, Saudi Arabia, and the Sultanate of Oman. Add the advent of three children to this hectic professional life and it is scarcely surprising that for many years George Hendry and this story were not uppermost in my mind.

Then, when I returned to Canada at the time of the first Gulf War and set up practice in Yarmouth, Nova Scotia, I read for the first time of George Hendry's carrying out an appendectomy on board HMCS *Ottawa* in Commander Tony German's superb history of the Canadian navy, *The Sea Is at Our Gates*. Finally, in 1999, I retired from practice and at last I could begin to tell the entire story.

This journey of search and research, writing and rewriting, has now spanned seven years. It has taken me to some widely disparate places, and on the way, I've met some wonderful and utterly unforgettable people. Now I want to recognize them and thank them.

Nearly all of the players, the people who knew and worked with George Hendry more than sixty-five years ago, are dead: my parents, all the doctors and nearly all the nurses, and all but a small handful of HMCS *Ottawa*'s surviving sailors. So it is a particular godsend that Carol Hendry Duffus, the senior surviving member of the Hendry family, George's biggest fan and favourite cousin, has such wonderfully clear memories of her "Uncle Will," George's father, William Belfry Hendry; of her "Aunt Bessie," George's mother, Elizabeth Robertson Hendry; of her two cousins, George's older brother, Jack, William John Hendry, and

George Ainslie Hendry himself. How often in the past seven years have I wished that I could raise some of these ghosts, just to talk with them!

I recall the many phone calls I had with the late Elizabeth Audrie ("Betty") Minogue, George Hendry's sweetheart and intended fiancée. Sweet, gentle, much-loved Betty died aged eighty-seven on April 10, 2006. I regret very much that I met this wonderful woman only once on an afternoon in Huntsville, Ontario, in late August 2001.

For the most part, there are no diaries and no dusty, forgotten boxes of letters. The letters went into the trash years ago and the diaries never got written. George Hendry had been cut down in his prime before he made his mark and before he could write many letters.

I am indebted to my cousin (and accomplished amateur genealogist), Ann Campbell Ward, RN, for conducting invaluable interviews on November 13, 2001, with Bernice Scott, RN, and Mildred Hall, RN, who were surviving TGH nursing classmates of George Hendry's wife, Jean Isobel Matthews, and who have since died. These two ladies, in turn, contacted several other of their nursing classmates of the class of 1938. Their memories and observations are included in Chapter Three.

There are at least thirty books on the Royal Canadian Navy during the Second World War, the Battle of the Atlantic, convoys, and anti-submarine warfare, covering both the men and their machines. Only five deal with the sinking of *Ottawa* and only two of these deal with this in any detail: Latham B. "Yogi" Jenson's superb book *Tin Hats, Oilskins and Seaboots: A Naval Journey 1938–45* and Tom Pullen's article "Convoy ON 127 & the Loss of HMCS *Ottawa*: A Personal Experience," published in the *Northern Mariner* in April 1992.

I will always be indebted to my dear friend, the late Yogi Jenson, and to the men who survived the sinking of *Ottawa* and shared their gripping first-hand stories, both those who have since passed on — Roe Skillen, Michael Barriault, Ed Fox, and George Johnson — and the five "doughty old salts" who live on today — Steve Logos, Sid Dobing, Al Underhill, Terry Terrabassi, and Norm Wilson. These were brave boys back then, along with all their other shipmates: I haven't had the honour of meeting them face to face, but I know them by the sound of their voices over the phone.

There are only four brief references to George Hendry's surgery, and only one of them describes the operations in any detail. The topic of wartime surgery on land is covered well in Bill Rawling's book *Death Their Enemy*, but surgery afloat has received almost no attention in published works.

Michael Whitby, the chief of the Naval History Team at the Directorate of Heritage and History at the Department of National Defence in Ottawa, was of absolutely indispensable assistance in making available through Library and Archives Canada the Reports of Proceedings (ROPs) for HMCS *St. Croix*, HMCS *Arvida*, and HMS *Celandine*, ships escorting convoy ON 127 in September 1942; the *Kriegstagebuch* (War Diary) of U-91; and the Records of Service for George Hendry, L.B. Jenson, T.C. Pullen, C.A. Rutherford, Dunn Lantier, and Lloyd Irwin Jones. ROPs and related memoranda for *Ottawa* from June 1938 to August 1942 were acquired through the Reference Services of Library and Archives Canada.

I could never have gained a fragment of the very necessary understanding of the *Ottawa* — the ship and its men — or the old Royal Canadian Navy and its contribution to victory in the Battle of the Atlantic without the wonderful advice and guidance given me by three people: Michael Whitby, Tony German, and the late Latham B. "Yogi" Jenson.

I would add my warm appreciation to others for encouragement and assistance: Bill Rawling, Naval History Team, Directorate of Heritage and History, Department of National Defence; Alma Jenson, Yogi Jenson's widow; Betty Pullen, Tom Pullen's widow; Kit Pullen, Tom Pullen's nephew; Captain (N) Dick Steele, RCN (Ret'd); Commander Fraser McKee, RCN (Ret'd); Commander Bob Rutherford, RCN (Ret'd); Stephen Kimber, King's College; Commodore H.A. "Mike" Cooper, RCN (Ret'd); Dr. Walter Hannah; J.G. Goodwin, QC; and, in Winchester (U.K.), Captain W.M. "Mike" Caswell, MVO, Royal Navy. I am most grateful for the considerable publication support extended by the Naval Officers Association of Canada through the good offices of its national president, Archdeacon Ronald E. Harrison.

I want now to thank some very special people who helped and encouraged me very considerably throughout this exhilarating seven years' journey: Michael Bliss, Professor Emeritus, University of Toronto; Dr. Tom Baskett, Professor of Gynaecology, Dalhousie University; Dr. Jock Murray, Dean of Medicine Emeritus, Dalhousie University; C. David Naylor, President, University of Toronto; Lennart Husband, University of Toronto

Press; Ani Orchanian-Chef, University Health Network Archives; Lagring Ulanday, Robarts Library, University of Toronto; Peter Shipp, Frank Shipp's eldest son; Susie Minogue and Peter Minogue, Betty Summers Minogue's daughter and son; Dr. Robert Meiklejohn; Jane Bryans; Leslie Ainger; Eleanor Wallbridge Lloyd; Dr. Bruce Thomas; Dr. Edwin Janke; Jodi Williamson, my last secretary; and computer guru extraordinaire Joe Doucette. I apologize if, in my dotage, I have inadvertently forgotten anybody.

Back at the beginning of this venture, my agent and my friend, the truly remarkable Elsa Franklin, asked me in that wonderfully direct way of hers, "Where are you going with this story?" So, just as the late Pierre Berton used to advise, I rewrote and rewrote this story six times until I felt it would hold the reader. I will always thank Elsa for that question.

I can't sufficiently thank the truly impressive people who make up The Dundurn Group for their great skill, their wisdom, and their patience in putting up with my infirmities: publisher Kirk Howard, editorial director Tony Hawke, editor Jennifer Gallant, and designer Alison Carr.

Finally, I owe more than can be said to my wife, Alison, my darling love and my best friend. She has not only confronted a debilitating illness with dignity and forbearance but has also tolerated my obsession with this book, my incessant talk of history, my absent-mindedness, and my absences with patience and cheerfulness. This is truly a gift.

Prologue:
A Burial at Sea

"Forasmuch as it hath pleased Almighty God of His great mercy to receive unto Himself the soul of our dear brother here departed: we therefore commit his body to the deep, looking for the resurrection of the body when the sea shall give up her dead..."

*T*he North Atlantic Ocean, five hundred miles east-northeast of Newfoundland. The late afternoon of Sunday, September 13, 1942. The quarterdeck of the Canadian destroyer HMCS *Ottawa*.

The ship's first lieutenant (executive officer), Lieutenant Thomas C. Pullen, is conducting "to the best of my ability ... a solemn burial service from the Book of Common Prayer."[1] Clustered around him are a group of perhaps thirty-five men. Some of them, the seamen of the destroyer ("ratings," or members of the "lower deck"), are turned out in their full dress uniforms — "number ones," or in Navy argot "pusser rig." There is also a group of men in rough working gear: pea jackets and dungarees. These are the rescued crew members of a torpedoed merchant ship, the tanker *Empire Oil.*

One of their number, a Royal Artillery marine gunner named Jones, has died this morning as a result of the excruciating abdominal injuries he received when the tanker was torpedoed three days ago. His body has been sewn into a canvas hammock and, following an ancient custom of the sea, the last stitch passed through the tip of the nose. A fifty-pound practice shell has been fixed between the legs to prevent the body from rising to the surface after being committed to the deep. The body in its canvas shroud has been laid out on a six-foot wooden plank, covered with a large White Ensign (the flag of the Royal Canadian Navy), and placed on a deck railing. An armed guard of honour consisting of an officer and eight men stands in a file on one side of the body.

The sky is a cheerless grey, but the sea is calmer than it has been for several days now. The ship is slipping along at ten knots, and the only sounds other than some voices are the hum of the ship's machinery and the gentle rippling of the bow wave. This scene is incongruously serene because the *Ottawa* is steaming five thousand yards ahead of the thirty-four-ship convoy that it is escorting in mid-Atlantic. The destroyer is one of six small warships scurrying around the convoy like sheepdogs safeguarding their flock from a marauding wolf pack of German U-boats. By this morning, these submarines have already sunk seven ships and seriously damaged four more. The one saving grace for the little *Ottawa* and its burial party is that U-boats make nearly all of their kills by attacking on the surface at night. So the service can proceed without much fear of interruption.

After the first lieutenant has read the service for burial at sea, the little bareheaded band sings the stirring old navy hymn:

> Eternal Father, strong to save,
> Whose arm hath bound the restless wave,
> Who bidd'st the mighty ocean deep
> Its own appointed limits keep:
> O hear us when we cry to Thee,
> For those in peril on the sea.

The honour guard then fires three volleys, six men hoist the plank, and the body slides from beneath the ensign into the sea. It has all been done by the book.[2]

Eight months after our declaration of war in early September 1939, a period of inactivity glibly dubbed the "phony war," we'd been rudely

22

shaken awake. First Norway and Denmark, then the Low Countries, and finally, in June 1940, France fell, leaving Britain isolated and alone. We were suddenly faced with the fact that the Mother Country (as our grandparents have called her for years) could survive only if it was successfully supplied by convoys across the North Atlantic.

German submarines trained as "wolf packs" by Grosadmiral Karl Dönitz could now sally forth from the newly captured ports on the Biscay coast of France to ambush our convoys. Winston Churchill calls this "the Battle of the Atlantic," and we are not ready to fight it. For the next two years, the number of merchant ships they sink vastly exceeds the number of U-boats we destroy. This is the "happy time" for German submariners.

Life in a wartime merchant ship on the North Atlantic is a lonely, cold, dirty, thankless, unglamorous, never-ending and very dangerous business. The speed of convoys making the run across to the United Kingdom and back is dictated by the slowest ship; all too frequently they travel at little more than six knots. If your munition ship is torpedoed, death is mercifully quick for everybody on board. If your tanker is hit, your end is slower. Either you burn in flaming oil or you choke to death breathing in the same stinking sludge on the water. Or, if you are just a little further north, you will probably die from immersion hypothermia in the Labrador Current.

Similarly, escorting convoys of merchant ships is a cold, wet, exhausting, dangerous, and decidedly unglamorous duty. It is the classic dirty job that somebody has to do, and we do it. We use older destroyers never intended to seek out and sink submarines and brand new corvettes purposely designed for this job.

Three days earlier, on September 10, the convoy had suddenly been ambushed by no less than thirteen German U-boats. At 1715 hours, soon after three other ships had been dispatched, the *Empire Oil*, a tanker of eight thousand tons sailing in ballast, was torpedoed, and the explosion blew a rivet deep into Gunner Jones's abdomen, tearing apart his intestine and causing him excruciating pain. The next day, *Ottawa's* doctor, Surgeon Lieutenant George Hendry, operated for nearly five hours in a valiant effort to save the poor man's life, patching up loop after loop of lacerated bowel. It was done, of necessity, on the small dining table of the captain's day cabin, as the ship's sick bay is little bigger than a closet.

Because there were four-metre seas, the patient had to be strapped down and Hendry had to depend on a bare minimum of the standard surgical instruments, crude ether anaesthesia given by the ship's sick berth attendant (SBA or "tiffy"), and willing but inexpert assistance from the first lieutenant and the destroyer's shipwright (carpenter).

Very few of the little group at poor Jones's burial service are true professionals. Less than half of the officers in the Royal Canadian Navy (RCN) trained in Royal Navy establishments overseas in the U.K. as cadets and midshipmen before the war. Others, the men of the Royal Canadian Naval Reserve (RCNR), "followed the seafaring life" with experience in the peacetime merchant marine.

Commodore Walter Hose, chief of the naval staff from 1921 to 1934, and the man many considered the father of the Royal Canadian Navy, created a sort of naval militia in communities right across the country and called it the Royal Canadian Naval Volunteer Reserve (RCNVR). Thus was born the "Wavy Navy," a nickname that arose from the undulating officers' rank stripes and gave birth to the sentimental wartime song "Roll along, Wavy Navy."

Up to one or two years ago, most joining the RCNVR have never been to sea at all. There is a popular wardroom jibe that holds that "the RCNVR are gentlemen trying to be officers, the RCNR are officers trying to be gentlemen, and the RCN are neither trying to be both."

There is one common factor, however. With few exceptions, the men are barely out of their teens. One of their number is Sub-Lieutenant Latham B. Jenson, the ship's twenty-one-year-old gunnery, signals, and radar officer. Jenson has been known as "Yogi" since his sea cadet days at home in Calgary before the war. He has already seen considerable action in several ships, large and small, and (by dint of passing promotion exams) just missed drowning with the 1,500-man crew of the famous battle cruiser HMS *Hood* when she blew up, hit by plunging shellfire from the German battleship *Bismarck*, on May 24, 1941. In later years, Yogi Jenson will record in writing and, through his remarkable talent as a naval artist, by illustration much of what happened to *Ottawa* during its last convoy run across the North Atlantic.[3]

The captain, Lieutenant Commander C.A. "Larry" Rutherford, remains constantly on the bridge conning the ship in its protective role ahead of the convoy. Aside from his gruelling performance in *Ottawa's* makeshift operating room, Surgeon Lieutenant George Hendry has worked through several nights tending to his two post-operative patients and patching up the other wounded sailors rescued from *Empire Oil.* Tom Pullen worried, "For the first time, I sensed that with the Captain, as with the Doctor, exhaustion was a matter for concern."[4]

The sad little burial service over, night falls and all is tranquil. The sea is calmer than it has been and the ship slips along at ten knots, five thousand yards ahead of the starboard wing of the convoy. A very faint blip on *Ottawa's* radar set is taken for a destroyer arriving from Newfoundland as a relief for the convoy's escort. Suddenly, at 2305, a tremendous explosion rocks the ship. A torpedo has blown the bow off. There is nothing forward of "B" gun but the sea. *Ottawa,* its engines stopped, lies dead in the water. Racing forward and clattering down a ladder into the "chaos and carnage," Tom Pullen finds the stokers' mess "transformed into a waist high jumble of damaged lockers, mess tables, hammocks, clothing, all framed by torn and twisted steel." Above him are "the bloody remains of lifeless men smashed upwards from their hammocks and impaled on overhead fittings by the tremendous force of the explosion."[5] To young Yogi Jenson, it resembles "a scene from hell."[6]

Then, at 2320, a second torpedo explodes into the number two boiler room with a huge flash and a "mind-numbing roar." The ship breaks in two, and what remains of the forward half of the ship heels to starboard and submerges rapidly. All of this takes place in seconds.

Last on the bridge, as the ship breaks up and rolls over, the captain and first lieutenant scramble down to the bilge keel. Then they jump in. Tom Pullen is weighed down by his waterlogged seaboots but manages to kick them off and surface. But the captain is gone. Utterly exhausted after four days on the bridge, he's given his lifebelt to a seaman who had none and has probably been dragged down by the waterlogged "lammy" (or duffel) coat he's been wearing.

Dr. George Hendry, too, is completely spent from six nearly sleepless days of operating, dressing wounds, and treating burns, on and on endlessly, right to the end. When the ship breaks up and begins sinking, he gets to a Carley float with some of the others and holds on. The wind and the sea flip this flimsy raft over and over again. George manages to get back and hold on three times, but the fourth time, he is so exhausted that he's just swept away in the dark.

Those who survive the sinking and the capsizing Carley floats have to contend with repeated jellyfish stings and the cold. However, even at its northern limit, the Gulf Stream is a few critical degrees warmer than its neighbour, the Labrador Current, and this happy fact undoubtedly saves many lives. Finally, after five hours in the sea, two corvettes from the convoy's escort group (HMS *Celandine* and HMCS *Arvida*) rescue sixty-nine men. But George Hendry is gone, along with 113 of his shipmates and 22 men rescued from *Empire Oil*. It has been a sad day and an awful night.

In a personal reminiscence written just before his untimely death fifty years later, Tom Pullen dubbed George Hendry "our gallant doctor,"[7] never knowing that long before that fatal night on the North Atlantic, there was another, darker side to this tragedy. It explains why he was carrying out this extraordinary surgery aboard a little destroyer in the North Atlantic and why he died out there. It accounts for his being in the navy in the first place.

George Hendry died when he was just thirty-one years old. His life spanned the Great War, the Roaring Twenties, and the Great Depression, and excepting summers spent on the Muskoka Lakes (and occasionally farther north when on a canoe trip with his brother, Jack) his world did not extend much beyond the environs of the city of Toronto. He'd never been overseas and had made only a very few trips outside Ontario. He had no connection at all with the Royal Canadian Navy. He'd never been to sea and, in fact, he'd never been on a ship of any size, unless you counted the little Muskoka steamers *Segwun* and *Sagamo* as ships. So when his death was announced, it must have come as quite a shock to his family and friends back home that he'd done some incredibly demanding major surgery on board a little destroyer before it was torpedoed in the middle of the North Atlantic.

And so, this story begins a very considerable distance from a spot out in the North Atlantic Ocean five hundred miles east-northeast of St. John's, Newfoundland.

The Hendrys:
A Remarkable Family

George Hendry was certainly not the conventional hero of the adventure novel having to scramble his way up from humble beginnings to accomplish great deeds or gain the ultimate position. True, George wasn't born with the proverbial silver spoon in his mouth, but he wanted for very little. He had wonderful, loving parents. He and his brother, Jack, were given a first-rate education at private schools. The family home in Toronto was substantial (but not ostentatious) and there was as well a summer house in Muskoka that was a treasured part of the family's life. The Hendrys were luckier than many of their neighbours in Toronto and a great many farmers in the West. They managed to survive the wild, roller-coaster ride first of the Roaring Twenties with its risky excesses and then the devastating ruin of the Dirty Thirties. Providentially, they got through the Great Depression relatively unscathed.

On March 24, 1939, George's father, William Belfry Hendry, the much revered professor emeritus of obstetrics and gynaecology in the University of Toronto's Faculty of Medicine, died at home after a year-long battle with leukaemia. To an impressive list of attributes covering his skill as a physician and a teacher and his wisdom, kindness, and integrity, my father added the following tribute: "He was the fortunate possessor of a boundless capacity for friendship and believed, with Emerson, that 'the only way to have a friend was to be one'."[8] Furthermore, he passed this immeasurable gift on to his sons.

Many of the professors (or "clinicians") who taught medical students and interns on the wards of Toronto's teaching hospitals during the twenties and thirties were colourful, utterly memorable characters and not at all fading violets. They seemed to jump right out of the pages of books like Richard Gordon's *Doctor in the House.* Some were lofty and aloof and suffered fools poorly. Some were adept and charming showmen, some bombastic, and others frankly eccentric. These men could arouse a kind of respect, even admiration on occasion, but nothing more. A few were humiliating bullies who made life a particular hell for students, interns, and junior staff and were hated for it.

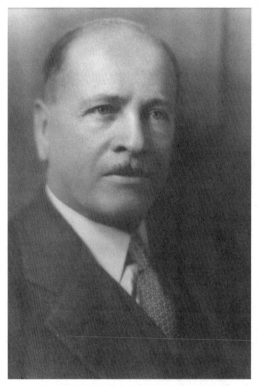

William Belfry Hendry, professor of obstetrics and gynaecology, University of Toronto, and obstetrician and gynaecologist-in-chief, Toronto General Hospital, 1922–36. To his colleagues young and old, he was always "the Chief." (Courtesy of Faculty of Medicine, Univeristy of Toronto.)

W.B. Hendry, on the other hand, was able to inspire loyalty, devotion, and deep affection in those he taught and those he worked with. That was his genius. William Osler might be worshipped by the people he trained.[9] Will Hendry was truly loved. To his colleagues, young and old, he was always known affectionately as "the Chief."

Nearly all the people of this story are dead, so it is a particular godsend that Carol Hendry Duffus, the senior surviving member of the Hendry family, has such wonderfully fond memories of her "Uncle Will," George's father, William Belfry Hendry; of her "Aunt Bessie," George's mother, Elizabeth Robertson Hendry; and of her two cousins, George's older brother

Jack, William John Hendry, and George Ainslie Hendry himself.

Carol's father, George M. Hendry, died mysteriously sometime after March 31, 1929,[10] just seven weeks after his second marriage, leaving Carol and her three sisters in the care of their emotionally unstable stepmother. When she proved incapable of this task, Uncle Will and Aunt Bessie brought their four young nieces more and more into their home in Toronto (286 Russell Hill Road) for dinners and other happy family gatherings, and brought them along on vacations at their cottage near Bala in the Muskoka district of Ontario. These memories have given us a priceless snapshot of the Hendry family during the Dirty Thirties.

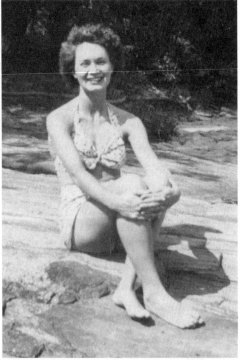

Carol Hendry, age twenty-four, was George's favourite cousin and greatest fan. This was taken during her last time at the Bala cottage, in August 1942. (Courtesy of Carol Hendry Duffus.)

During his undergraduate days at the University of Toronto, Will Hendry was an outstanding athlete, winning university colours in rugby, soccer, lacrosse, and gymnastics. After taking a Bachelor of Arts degree in 1895 and attending teachers' college (the Ontario School of Pedogogy), he taught mathematics for three years at Ridley College. However, this was not the career he had in mind for himself, and so he entered Toronto's Faculty of Medicine and graduated MB (Medicinae Baccalaureus, or Bachelor of Medicine, the degree granted at the time) in 1904. There is a particularly delightful photograph of a group of young doctors at the old Burnside Lying-in Hospital, each holding a newborn baby. Some appear nonchalant and some seem very self-conscious. Only Will Hendry seems genuinely involved, and he has a wonderful smile on his face.

In those days, most young graduate physicians would go straight into general practice, without doing an internship. A very few would go on to take postgraduate training: if they could afford it, they would go to Great Britain, Germany, or even to the United States. Otherwise they got this sort of experience at home. Will Hendry did just that and spent the next two years as a house surgeon at the old Toronto General Hospital on Gerrard Street. In 1906 he was appointed a junior demonstrator in the university's Department of Obstetrics and Gynaecology, and by 1912 he was an assistant professor.

W.B. Hendry had an early start in the military as a private in the Canadian Army Medical Corps (CAMC; the prefix "Royal" came much later) during his medical school days in 1901. By the time that war was declared in August 1914, he was a major; by May 1915 he was on his way overseas as a lieutenant colonel and second-in-command of # 4 Canadian General Hospital. This unit was ordered to Salonika in November 1915 to support the British forces on the Greco-Macedonian front.[11] He was appointed to command the hospital in January 1917 and was promoted full colonel in December of that year. For meritorious service, he was twice Mentioned in Despatches and was decorated with the Distinguished Service Order (DSO) by King George V.

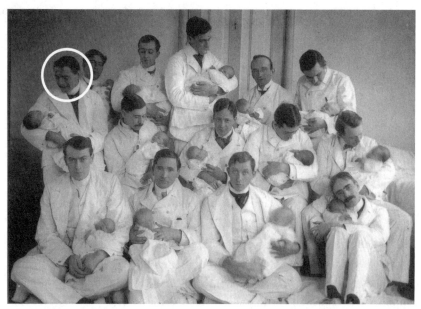

W.B. Hendry (circled) in a group of interns at Toronto General Hospital in 1904, each holding a very young patient. He's obviously enjoying this task far more than his fellow housemen, most of whom are looking either terrified or studiously nonchalant. (Courtesy of Carol Hendry Duffus.)

W.B. Hendry returned to civilian life in July 1919 after serving more than four years overseas. In 1922, he was appointed professor of obstetrics and gynaecology in the University of Toronto and obstetrician and gynaecologist-in-chief at the Toronto General Hospital. In the fourteen years to follow, he built up a truly outstanding university department.

After his death in March 1939, the resolution passed by the faculty council stated that "he counted it his greatest achievement that he had been able to foster the careers of a large number of his younger colleagues,"[12] one of them being my father.

On March 25, 1928, my dad, then a twenty-five-year-old obstetrical house surgeon (resident) at TGH, wrote in his journal, "The Prof. [W.B. Hendry] came down to my room ... & offered me an opportunity of going in with him and sharing his office & also to pay me an honorarium of $600 per year for assisting him with operations, etc.... He offered me a Junior Demonstratorship in the University Department and a part-time research fellowship."[13]

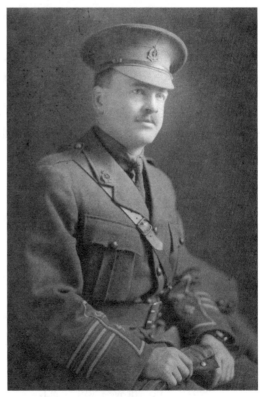

Thus began what proved to be a much-valued professional relationship over the next ten years: first as assistant and mentor, and then as colleagues and close friends.

The resolution passed by the faculty council after my father's death in 1953 stated that "his association with Dr. Hendry soon became one of mutual admiration and friendship, a relationship which was greatly treasured by Dr. Goodwin and which profoundly affected his professional life."[14]

In 1930, Drs. Hendry and Goodwin moved into 516

Lieutenant Colonel W.B. Hendry, Commanding Officer, Number 4 Canadian General Hospital, Salonika, Greece, 1916. (Courtesy of Carol Hendry Duffus.)

Medical Arts Building, an office my father occupied for the next twenty years and subsequently shared with George Hendry when he had completed his postgraduate training. Carol Hendry Duffus recalls:

> During the time that Uncle Will was ill and failing, I spent quite a bit of time with him. I remembered all the times we had been together, looking at him at the dining-room table, noticing his yellow moustache & stained teeth and fingers from smoking too much. I always wondered if that was the reason he was ill.[15] We became close and he told me many tales of his life. I'd never realized he had been away so long during WWI or that he had received the DSO or that he was so well respected by his associates. He was just my uncle! I learned all of this much later on.

Carol's "Uncle Will" married "Aunt Bessie," Elizabeth Robertson McMichael, in 1907. By all accounts, she and Will had a good marriage. She was bright, set high standards for their two sons, and was a very loving mother. She was, Carol says, "a quiet woman, not very active. I never saw her swim: she had asthma and difficulty breathing. She wheezed so loudly, that sometimes I thought there was a cat in the room! … As I grew older, I became more aware of who she was. She'd suddenly quote poetry or share an opinion and I realized how well read and knowledgeable she was."

Elizabeth Hendry kept what she called a "diary" of both her sons written after their deaths, although it was really a rather ornate history. She devoted eighteen pages to Jack but only two to George. At first blush, this might suggest a tinge of favouritism, but she rejects this emphatically: "As the two boys grew older, their lives became very closely interwoven, and the story of one is the story of the other."

William John Hendry, "Jack to all who knew and loved him," was born on October 28, 1909.

> He showed ability early. He walked at nine months and began to talk at quite an early age…. He astonished us all on one occasion by reading the names on the street-cars and distinguishing the various car lines….

Whatever Jack did, he did it well.... His power of concentration was developed to a marked degree. Figures had a fascination for him and later he showed evidence of a brilliant mathematical mind. Later, too, his interest in science developed....

All through his life, Jack showed evidence of reasoning powers much beyond the average.

George Ainslie Hendry was born on February 4, 1911, and "was a very delicate child." During the war years particularly, "the boys suffered from various childhood illnesses. George seemed to suffer more than Jack. When both developed measles, Jack had no complications, but George developed pneumonia and middle ear trouble, and was really a very sick little lad."

In 1912, the Hendrys bought a cottage (or "house" as Elizabeth calls it in her diary) on Struan Point near Bala on Lake Muskoka. For the next thirty years, this place was a treasured part of Hendry family life.[16]

George was barely four years old when his father went overseas in May 1915. For the next four years until Will returned, Elizabeth Hendry and her sister, Jean McMichael, were the boys' parents. Jack used to tell amused neighbours that he had "one daddy and two mothers." During the war years, Elizabeth did volunteer work with the Red Cross in Toronto and in Bala.

The boys' "happiest memories circled around their Muskoka days." From 1912 onwards, every summer was spent at Bala. "Very early, the boys learned to swim.... Both became excellent swimmers and divers, and were able to handle a canoe admirably."

George steadily overcame his health problems and, by the time his father came home from the Great War, he was well on his way to becoming a superb athlete. One suspects that there were somewhat stronger ties between George and his dad because of the father's enthusiasm for and achievement in sport.

Northern Ontario is some of the best canoe-tripping country in the world, and each summer from 1923 to 1927 the Hendry boys and friends took full advantage of this fact with longer and more demanding trips from Muskoka to the Magnetawan, Algonquin Park, Lake Nipissing, and Temagami.

Carol Hendry Duffus has happy memories of summers at the Bala cottage during the thirties:

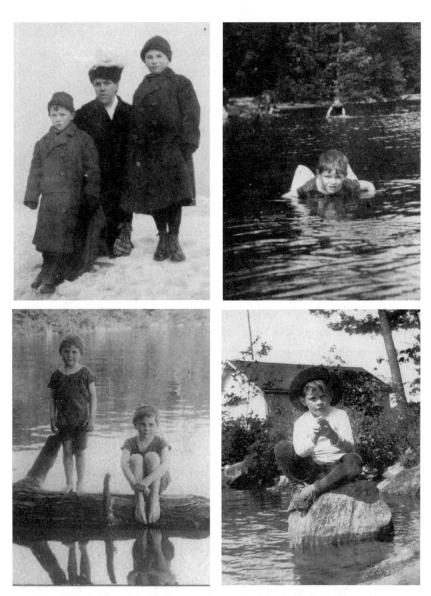

Top left: Elizabeth Robertson Hendry ("Aunt Bessie") with her boys in winter 1916 — George, age five, and Jack, age seven — while their father is overseas commanding a Canadian General Hospital in Macedonia. Top right: George, age seven, swimming at the Bala "house" in the summer of 1918. Bottom left: The Hendry boys on a log at Bala, Lake Muskoka, in the summer of 1916. Bottom right: George Hendry, age seven (summer 1918), in a cove behind the Bala cottage boathouse, looking rather like a Canadian Tom Sawyer. (Courtesy of Carol Hendry Duffus.)

It wasn't too happy a place on the home front, as you know, so my sisters and I would look forward to the summer when Uncle Will and Aunt Bessie asked us to Bala for part of it. George usually picked us up and drove us. If he hated the job, he certainly never showed it and made us welcome and loved to tease us with his driving technique. He always got a rise out of us, especially when coming to the brow of a hill, he'd drop down the other side, leaving us squealing with our stomachs in our throats.

George was studying to be a doctor like his older brother Jack. He was to specialize in obstetrics and gynaecology later. He had a way with kids and would have made a good paediatrician, too. He was in Toronto during the week studying or interning and we'd look forward to the weekends when he and Jack all came to swell the numbers. We'd caddy for the men, go on picnics, pick berries, swim and boat. It was wonderful. George was a good teacher — a fine athlete and paddler. He taught me canoe handling and later to drive the beautiful "Muskoka" boat with the inboard motor.

On many occasions, he'd bring one or two of his close friends up — all future doctors — Frank Shipp, Hank Swan were two I remember — and they'd include us girls. It was the era of the "Big Bands" and many of those came to perform at Dunn's in Bala. What a great time we had!

No one could have had a better cousin: so kind, thoughtful and giving, and with such a great sense of humour. From what we heard over the years, he was a very popular and well liked person — morally good to the core. I certainly agree with all of that because I knew him for many years.

Both Jack and George were sent to the Model School (an institution in East Toronto now long defunct) and then in 1921 to University of Toronto Schools (UTS) on Bloor Street West. By that time, the Hendrys had moved to 154 Walmer Road, just three blocks north of UTS, which made easy walking for the boys. In 1920, "or thereabouts," Jack was struck with diphtheria complicated by myocarditis, which took him out of school for four months of bed rest at home. His mother told how the "long period of inaction due to his illness influenced his attitude toward sport. Jack never became very proficient, whilst George was constantly busy with games; hockey, football, baseball." At UTS, "Jack's learning and George's ability in football and hockey were much in evidence."

In his first three years at UTS, Jack Hendry skipped one year and won four scholarships. When he matriculated in 1926, he won thirteen first-class honours and four more scholarships, all before he was seventeen.

No record survives of George's scholastic achievements at UTS, but he clearly acquitted himself well enough to gain admission into medical school. The *Twig*, the school journal, reported some of his athletic accomplishments:

- 1924: "outstanding skill and ability on the Gym Team."
- 1926: "G.A. Hendry played outside on the 120 lb. Rugby Team."
- 1927: "the 120 lb. Rugby Team was led by Hendry…. Good things come in small packages." (George was just 5' 8".)
- 1928: "Hendry was a goal-getter in Midget Hockey."
- 1929 (Alumni News): "Hendry has been practising with the Varsity Junior Hockey Team" in his first year in Medicine at University of Toronto.

Toronto, the city that George Hendry grew up in, was staid, righteous, conservative (small and large "c"), Protestant (Anglican, Orange Order, etc.), and resolutely British. Indeed, Toronto was probably the most British city in Canada: 85 percent of its population could claim British ancestry. Another 6 percent were Jewish, and among the remainder were Italians, Greeks, Macedonians, Chinese, and Blacks. We were too proud of our "Britishness," and this undoubtedly created a class structure that isolated us. The resulting prejudice and racism was accepted almost as a matter of course. Jews were denied admission to hotels and restricted from membership in clubs and organizations. Few Jewish students were enrolled in Toronto's medical school and the university's teaching hospitals appointed no Jewish doctors to their staffs. This disturbing state of affairs persisted until well after the Second World War.[17]

In the aftermath of the Russian Revolution of October 1917, there was a pervasive fear of anarchy, Bolshevism, and the flood of "undesirables" from Eastern Europe. Because of the Mother Country's high standard of morality, our very Britishness led inexorably to prejudice, racism, and xenophobia. And so on to a federal ban on immigration, vicious police suppression of communists, and calls for eugenic sterilization of the feeble-minded in order to stop the spread of insanity, alcoholism, moral degeneration, and so-called "pauperism."

The conviction that unbridled immigration and promiscuity led to the genetic transmission of feeble-mindedness prompted a host of public-spirited Alberta women (including Emily Murphy of the "Famous Five," who, in 1929, managed to have women legally acknowledged as "persons") to campaign forcefully and successfully in 1928 for the passage of the now infamous Sexual Sterilization Act of the Province of Alberta. In 1933, the very year that Nazi leader Adolf Hitler came to power in Germany, Herbert Bruce, the eminent surgeon and lieutenant-governor of Ontario, spoke grandiloquently of the "racial degeneration" and "moral perversion" resulting from "unchecked propagation" of the mentally defective. Dr. Bruce recommended with no little heat that this "evil" be "stamped out" by wholesale sterilization.[18] Even though this sort of legislation was never considered in Ontario, third-year medical students in Toronto at the time were offered an elective course in "human heredity and eugenics."[19]

Ontario took a different tack than Alberta to deal with the vexing problem of moral degeneration. It resorted to a brutal regulation called the Female Refuge (not "refug<u>ee</u>") Act of 1897 to bring down the full weight of the law on poor teenage girls considered to be "dissolute" or "promiscuous." In 1939, one such unfortunate, Velma Demerson — eighteen years old, single, and pregnant — was arrested, charged with being "incorrigible," and sentenced to one year in Toronto's infamous Mercer Reformatory for Females. Like a character in a Dickens or a Brontë novel, she endured long hours working in the reformatory's sewing factory, the strictest discipline, spartan food, numerous degrading pelvic examinations, excruciatingly painful treatment for vaginal warts without anaesthesia, weeks of solitary confinement, and, finally, the apprehension of her newborn child by the state. Her crime? She had had the temerity to fall in love and so "consort" with a Chinese man. After her imprisonment, she married her lover and, as a final indignity, lost her citizenship for some years as a result.[20] There were many other examples of similar gothic horrors in this place until it was closed and torn down in 1969.

Though not as recklessly as our neighbour to the south, Toronto was carried away with the good times of the Roaring Twenties — the social liberation, the constant pursuit of pleasure and profit, the boom before the bust of the Dirty Thirties. To resist these excesses, "Toronto the Good" had to be morally vigilant at all times. The family honour was sacrosanct; professional reputation was everything. Scandal was anathema. The discoverer of insulin, Frederick Banting, went through a messy and very public divorce in 1932, and the Empire was badly shaken by the abdication of King Edward VIII in favour of the twice-divorced Mrs. Simpson in 1936.

Toronto was a city of churches, mostly Protestant churches. Eighty-five percent of Torontonians were Protestants, the majority Anglicans and the remainder Methodists, Presbyterians and Congregationalists (who combined as the United Church of Canada in 1928), and Baptists. In response to the so-called Blue Laws,[21] everything (except the churches) closed down on Sunday: stores, restaurants, theatres, movie houses, sports events, and, of course, all the bars. You couldn't buy a stick of gum. It used to be said that you could fire a gun down Yonge Street on Sunday and never hit a thing. We were indeed WASPs — White, Anglo-Saxon Protestants — and the acronym stuck.

For Toronto, "that maiden aunt of cities,"[22] the decade 1919–1929 was a time of burgeoning, liberating, bewildering change: architectural masterpieces like Union Station, the Royal York Hotel, and Eaton's College Street store sprang up; motor cars pushed the horse gradually out to pasture; living conditions immeasurably improved as slums like "the Ward" were cleared; children were dying less often with communicable diseases like tuberculosis, scarlet fever, and diphtheria; women were surviving childbirth with better obstetric care; the iceman was being replaced by the electric refrigerator; young women were emancipated — they bobbed their hair, shortened their skirts, rolled down their stockings, started smoking, and now could vote; men wore hats to work and suits with vests; gentlemen wore top hats to the races and spats to board meetings; there were talking movies at Loews or Shea's Hippodrome; couples danced to the music of Luigi Romanelli at the King Edward Hotel; the sale of alcohol was first banned and then controlled; bridge and mah-jong were all the rage; every August until Labour Day, the whole family went to the "Ex," the Canadian National Exhibition. This was certainly the Roaring Twenties, and we seemed to inherit most of it from the United States of America.

Very slowly, the city began to recover from the awfulness and the grief of what people called "the war to end all wars." From a population of well under half a million, it had sent an astounding seventy thousand of its men to the trenches in France and Flanders. Of Canada's sixty thousand "glorious dead," thirteen thousand were Toronto boys; many more were left maimed and permanently disfigured. Though many of the returning "rankers" might not be sure about what they had fought for, they began to realize that Canada was on a more equal footing with the Mother Country. The men who came home held on to their sense of duty and loyalty to the Crown. We ecstatically endorsed this love of monarchy during three Royal Tours across Canada — two by the immensely popular Prince of Wales in 1919 and 1927, the third by King George VI and Queen Elizabeth in 1939. David Windsor's abdication in 1936 as King Edward VIII in favour of the twice-divorced Wallis Warfield Simpson certainly jolted the Empire, but it did little to erode our allegiance to the Mother Country.

In those days, we honoured the men who had fallen in the Great War, speaking reverently of their "devotion to duty" and their "supreme sacrifice." This was inextricably linked to patriotism and allegiance to the Crown. Men like Will Hendry believed in these things instinctively, but they didn't go around spreading the word like pious, moralizing evangelists. It was entirely a private matter.

Men returning to their peacetime professions (physicians, especially) in the aftermath of the Great War retained their strong sense of duty, honour, service, and sacrifice. They considered that the development of these values was the *sine qua non* in the building of character in their sons. In those days, daughters were to be protected rather than prepared. This was the stuff and staple of private schools all over the Empire, like Brookfield in James Hilton's novella, *Goodbye, Mr. Chips.* The long honour rolls in their prayer halls carried the names (in gold leaf) of old boys who had given their lives in the exercise of these virtues at Ypres, the Somme, Vimy, and Passchendaele. A long-forgotten poem by Sir Henry Newbolt, "*Vitai Lampada*," epitomizes these qualities. It was a very popular recitation during and after the Great War:

> There's a breathless hush in the Close tonight —
> Ten to make and the match to win —
> A bumping pitch and a blinding light,
> An hour to play and the last man in.
> And it's not for the sake of a ribboned coat,
> Or the selfish hope of a season's fame,
> But his Captain's hand on his shoulder smote —
> "Play up! play up! and play the game!"
>
> The sand of the desert is sodden red, —
> Red with the wreck of a square that broke; —
> The Gatling's jammed and the Colonel dead,
> And the regiment blind with dust and smoke.
> The river of death has brimmed his banks,
> And England's far, and Honour a name,
> But the voice of a schoolboy rallies the ranks:
> "Play up, play up, and play the game!"

This was expected to stir schoolboys then and it did.

In late September 1926, Jack Hendry entered the four-year Biology and Medical Sciences (B&M) course, and with his characteristically quiet excellence, he graduated with first-class honours in June 1930, second in his year. His passage through the three years of the undergraduate course in medicine was similarly distinguished. This remarkable young man was elected a member of AOA (Alpha Omega Alpha) honour medical fraternity, was the associate editor of the *University of Toronto Medical Journal*, and had managed to take the Edward Blake Scholarship, the Dunlap Scholarship in Psychiatry twice, and the War Memorial Scholarship twice. At graduation in June 1933, he won the Gold Medal in Medicine, standing first overall in his year, and was awarded the prestigious Ellen Mickle Fellowship, which enabled him to take up a research appointment in reproductive endocrinology with Dr. Carl Hartman at the Carnegie Institution in Baltimore.

He began work in Baltimore on September 26, 1933, and, as might have been predicted, impressed everyone working at the Carnegie with his acuteness of mind, his phenomenal memory, and his capacity for friendship. As his mother tells us, Dr. Hartman was so pleased with the work that Jack had done on a paper to do with their research that he asked him to present the paper himself to a group of senior colleagues in New York later that year.

On February 6, 1934, while working in the institution's vivarium, Jack was bitten by a monkey. At first he was thought to have developed "intestinal grippe," but "for comfort's sake" he was admitted to the Johns Hopkins Hospital on February 15. Then the symptoms began to look like those seen with classic poliomyelitis, and, quite suddenly, he took a turn for the worse. By the time his father, mother, and brother got there, it was too late. He'd gone into respiratory paralysis; there was nothing to be done for him "and so he left us."

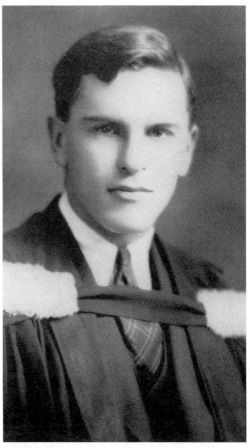

The tributes poured in. This was a much-loved young man. Not only was he gifted and brilliant but he was also good, kind, modest to a fault, and possessed of quiet strength. His memory would serve as an inspiration to all. Emil Novak, the internationally famous gynaecological pathologist in later years, wrote to Jack's parents, "How much your boy was admired and loved by all with whom he came in contact. I am truthful when I say that I can think of no young man who had made a finer impression than Jack and no one who was more generally loved."

William John ("Jack") Hendry at graduation from the University of Toronto Faculty of Medicine in June 1933, age twenty-three. (Courtesy of Carol Hendry Duffus.)

In the end, Elizabeth Hendry's diary survives as a well-written testament to her dead sons. There is no doubt that she loved George.

She had worshipped Jack, but Jack was gone.

Now it was George's turn to shine.

The Making of a Doctor:
G.A. Hendry, Meds 3T5

George Hendry's education as a doctor and his postgraduate training as an obstetrician coincided exactly with the Great Depression.[23] For Torontonians, this worst peacetime calamity of the twentieth century began in earnest (after a number of false starts) on Black Tuesday, October 29, 1929, at the Stock Exchange on Bay Street in downtown Toronto and ended with the declaration of the Second World War on September 3, 1939.

In three years, stocks depreciated a catastrophic 85.7 percent, from a 1929 high of $6,265,709,154 to a 1932 low of $880,229,083. By May 1, 1933, 32.1 percent (or nearly one in three) of the national workforce was unemployed, and 1.5 million people (15 percent of the population of Canada) were on relief ("pogey" or "the dole"). In 1931, rural schoolteachers' salaries were slashed from $1,100 to $780, and they were paid in notes that the banks would refuse to cash.[24]

Thousands lost their life savings, dozens of banks closed, farm mortgages foreclosed like falling dominoes, a pervasive drought with failed crops swept across Western Canada, and two prime ministers (first Mackenzie King and then R.B. Bennett) completely misjudged the gravity of this economic tsunami.

In a letter to Prime Minister R.B. Bennett on January 14, 1935, a man in Galahad, Alberta, suggested a creative solution for the unemployment problem: "First I would suggest a method or a law, whereby Females would not be allowed employment as long as a Male can fill that or those posissions. [*sic*] ... If the young men were in these posissions they would be able to support a wife, therefore would increase Population & so we would not have so much unemployment."[25]

Anything smacking of communism and its trappings was blamed for this disaster, and innocent bystanders who strayed into the midst of a protest were beaten, charged, and thrown into jail. The Russian Revolution had occurred just twelve years ago, and it was only two years since Sacco and Vanzetti had been unjustly executed for murder in the United States because they were held to be anarchists. Canada was British to the core and "foreigners," that is anyone not having compelling ties to the United Kingdom, were almost automatically suspect.

The city of Toronto had indulged in a spate of grand building construction, barely in time to avoid the crash. In 1927, the hugely popular Prince of Wales had opened the magnificent new Union Station and had dedicated the Prince's Gate at the Canadian National Exhibition. This was followed in 1929 by the Royal York Hotel, the largest of its kind in the British Empire. Not to be outdone, the Bank of Commerce added the tallest skyscraper in the Empire. Eaton's then contributed its architecturally chic art deco store on College Street, a block east of the site of the Private Patients Pavilion, a much-needed addition to the Toronto General Hospital. The construction of the splendid new Private Patients Pavilion was begun just before Black Tuesday in October 1929 and was finished in record time in April 1930. And then, in 1931, when the Depression's full effect was being felt, the workers who put up Maple Leaf Gardens, the "house that Connie Smythe built," were paid in shares in lieu of wages.

True, Toronto hadn't been hit as hard as the West, but it certainly did suffer.

Within a month of the crash, 10,000 were out of work in the city; one morning, 347 hungry men were counted lining up for a meal outside the Scott Mission. There came a steady stream of unemployed men into the "good" residential neighbourhoods, and a surprising number of those who knocked on doors asking for a handout, a castoff overcoat, or a meal were well-educated, middle-class professionals. Though no record remains of their financial situation, the Hendry family was certainly not destitute. Nevertheless, people left with sufficient resources and some security in that awful time didn't have to look far for others who had lost everything.

In the late 1930s, I can remember the returned soldiers from the Great War, most of whom were still on the sunny side of fifty, parading at the CNE Grandstand, and they could even manage to trot out a little group of survivors of the Boer War of 1899–1902, the old "Soldiers of the Queen"! It was only a scant eleven years or so since the Great War, and in spite of crippling unemployment among returned soldiers, Toronto continued to be unswervingly British. There was a sign hung in an East London street during the Silver Jubilee celebrations for King George V and Queen Mary that stated proudly "POOR BUT LOYAL."[26] This sentiment was equally applicable to Canadians in that trying time. Patriotism was not debatable in 1935.

Dr. Herbert A. Bruce, the lieutenant-governor of Ontario (and the renowned surgeon who founded the Wellesley Hospital in Toronto), sent the following comments in an urgent letter to Prime Minister R.B. Bennett on August 10, 1934:

> There are certainly not less than 1500 houses [in Toronto] that are unhealthy…. There are certain districts, notably from the Don River to Dovercourt and south of College and Carleton Streets which … may be termed blighted areas…. In these districts, the defects of the environment often make unsatisfactory even those houses that are in good condition.
>
> Satisfactory houses for families of average size cost at least $25.00 to $30.00 per month, while many employed heads of families can pay no more than $15.00 to $20.00. [27]

Just how sick (or how well) were we Torontonians in the Dirty Thirties? Right at the top of the list of health concerns for both doctors and the public were children's communicable diseases like scarlet fever, whooping cough, diphtheria, poliomyelitis ("infantile paralysis"), tuberculosis, meningitis, and pneumonia. Infectious disease was the number one killer of both children and adults at that time. There were no real antibiotics as we know them. Alexander Fleming had just accidentally uncovered the in vitro antibacterial properties of *penicillium notatum* mold, but any practical usefulness was still years away. Immunization and vaccination were the only therapies. "Hygiene" was the byword of medical practice. Houses were quarantined (from the Italian *quaranta*: forty) for up to forty days or more for the more contagious of these diseases. Relatives, visitors,[28] and tradesmen were warned away by a sinister placard placed by order in a front window of the house.

The Ontario infantile paralysis epidemic of August–September 1937 produced 2,546 cases of poliomyelitis and 119 deaths. A panic ensued ("Do something! Do anything!"[29]); the public and the doctors grasped at straws. Because of promising results reported in Alabama, the prophylactic use of zinc sulphate nasal spray was advocated to cauterize the nerve sheaths in the roof of the nasal passages and thus prevent the transmission of polio virus into the brain. On August 31, 1937, 5,233 children were sprayed, and two weeks later, 4,585 children were sprayed a second time. By November 1937, a number of these children had lost (at least temporarily) their sense of smell and in any event the spray had been shown to be totally ineffective.

There was, however, one significant ray of sunshine. While all of this haphazard and panicky activity was being played out, Robert Defries and J.G. Fitzgerald at the University of Toronto's School of Hygiene and the Connaught Laboratories developed the world's first effective immunizing toxoid for that other killer of children, diphtheria.

Cancer was treated carelessly with crude radiotherapy and inadequate surgery. It was diagnosed too late, and early screening methods like Pap smears were unheard of. Many specialists prepared and administered their own radium in their offices or else without adequate protection on open hospital wards. In 1932, after considerable political wrangling, the Toronto General Hospital purchased a quantity of radium, and the Ontario Radiotherapy Institute was opened in the old Dunlap Pathology Laboratory building.

Coronary artery disease and hypertension were not taken too seriously and frequently took second place to the treatment of chronic rheumatic heart disease. Endocrinology was just emerging as a subspecialty with obvious advances in the treatment of diabetes and thyroid disease.

Even as late as the mid-thirties in Toronto,[30] more than half of all pregnant women still gave birth at home, and in rural communities the figure was close to 100 percent. Indeed, senior U of T medical students got their obstetrical experience by delivering babies in the patients' homes. Across Ontario in 1935, 530 women died in childbirth for every 100,000 live births! This statistic is called the maternal mortality ratio, and nowadays in Canada it stands at 6. These women died with the convulsions and cerebral haemorrhages of pregnancy toxaemia, with fulminating puerperal infections (for which there were no effective antibiotics) as a result of illegal backstreet abortions, and with uncontrolled postpartum haemorrhaging (for which there were no safe blood transfusions).

Statistics from the Burnside Hospital (the public obstetrical wing of TGH) showed that premature newborns rarely survived if they weighed less than three pounds at birth. Concern for preemies was only a glimmer on the horizon, and the concept of regionalization of perinatal care, with systematic communication between caregivers and consultants and rapid dependable transport, was unheard of. Accordingly, it is nothing short of miraculous that on the morning of May 28, 1934, in the little Northern Ontario community of Corbeil, all five of the Dionne quintuplets survived some pretty crude management techniques and, equally incredible, twenty-five-year-old Mrs. Elzire Dionne (who had already delivered five children) did not succumb to frighteningly severe toxaemic hypertension and postpartum haemorrhage.[31]

During twelve days in July 1936, a catastrophic heat wave hit Ontario and parts of eastern Manitoba: 1,180 people died, and of these 400 drowned seeking relief from the heat. On the sixth day, the death toll in Ontario had reached 458. "More than 220 dead in Toronto," exclaimed the *Toronto Daily Star.*[32] Air conditioning was a technology off in the future and canvas awnings over windows of their houses offered only partial relief for people with money.

In those days, your health care depended on your ability to pay. If you had a good job or if your family had money, you could afford a specialist, a private room in the new Private Patients Pavilion, and probably a "private duty nurse." Newly graduated nurses could make a modest living in the Depression attending private post-operative or postpartum cases. Women frequently remained in a hospital bed for two and sometimes three weeks after having a baby in those days.

If you were out of work, on relief, or just poorly paid, you'd have to be seen at one of the outpatient (or "outdoor") clinics in the city when you were sick. If you needed to come into hospital for something serious like pneumonia or surgery, you'd be admitted to one of those long, cavernous, drafty, forty-bed public wards in the College Street Building of the Toronto General Hospital. In the screened-off bed next to you, some poor old fellow might die in the night but the curtains around the bed on the other side couldn't keep out the smell of an enema or the moaning of an unsedated patient. For imminent childbirth you'd be sent to the old Burnside "Lying-in" (meaning obstetrical) Hospital.

Doctors in Ontario were paid for services to indigent people on what was called "medical relief" according to the following fee schedule: office visit, $2.00; home visit, $3.00; maternity care, $25.00.

The Ontario Department of Public Welfare and Municipal Affairs (not the Department of Health) paid physicians thirty-five cents per month per person on medical relief. The gross account was paid monthly to the doctor, not in full but in proportion to the funds available to that department. Six cents of the monthly allotment of thirty-five cents was reserved for drugs.[33]

So, you were either a "private" patient or a "public" patient. This sort of social stratification refused to die until well after the Second World War, as illustrated by the following incident: One morning many years ago, a lowly junior intern (that's what they called us then) at the Toronto Western Hospital was presenting a patient's case to a gathering of his peers and masters at what was called (grandly enough) "grand rounds": "This fifty-four-year-old lady was admitted with cough, fever, weight loss...." That's as far as he got, because the venerable chief of the medical service interrupted: "Doctor, you should be saying: 'This fifty-four-year-old woman.' This is the Public Ward."

On Tuesday morning, September 24, 1929, exactly five weeks before the bottom fell out of Wall Street and Bay Street, George Hendry registered as a first-year student of medicine at the University of Toronto. As was and always has been the custom at "Varsity," he was now forever linked to his year of graduation as a member of "Meds 3T5."

The University of Toronto had (and has) the best medical school in Canada. In those long-ago days, most of the professors — the teachers of both the basic science and the practice of medicine — were indelible and unforgettable characters. Toronto's medical students worked hard and played hard. A host of colourful stories have survived.

Most graduating physicians went into general practice, frequently in small country towns from which they rarely returned. A few stayed on to train as specialists in the big city and a very few pursued pure research.

The world of Toronto's university and its medical school that George Hendry had entered on that Tuesday morning was not entirely foreign to him. His father was its professor of obstetrics and gynaecology and his brother was already a student of medicine there.

The annual fee for the first year, "including tuition, library, laboratory supply and one annual examination," was $150, "payable at the Bursar's office in Simcoe Hall between the hours of ten and one o'clock, except on Saturday." The fee for the second through sixth years jumped to $200 to include the fee for "one session's clinical teaching facilities at the Toronto General Hospital, St. Michael's Hospital, or Toronto Western Hospital and the Hospital for Sick Children, but does not cover the midwifery ticket for the Burnside Lying-in Hospital, which must be paid in addition, to the Bursar."[34, 35] (This is in stark contrast to the galactic $14,000 tuition imposed at the University of Toronto in 2000–01![36])

Like his father and brother, George had an enormous capacity for making and keeping friends — Henry Swan, Art Squires, and Herb Tait among many. His best friend was certainly Frank Loudon Shipp, both his classmate and teammate on the Senior OHA hockey team, of which George was captain in 1934.

At graduation, his medical class numbered one hundred men and eight women. It turned out to be a distinguished class: one university president, two medical school deans, five department chairmen, not a few senior professors, and several outstanding clinicians. A.L. Chute, A.H. Squires, J.D. Hamilton, H.M.S. Tait, J.C. McKellar, and Marjorie Davis were those of George's classmates whom I knew in the fifties and sixties and beyond.

Training to be a doctor was (and still is) like any other rite of passage. You had to crawl before you stand, stand before you walk, walk before you run, and so on up the hill. Thus, the medical student first mastered the traditional preclinical disciplines like anatomy and pathology. Then he learned how to link what he had learned in anatomy lab and looking down a microscope with the patient's disease process, how to take a history and do a physical examination, how to listen with a stethoscope, and how to write a prescription. At last, he got on to a hospital ward or into a clinic as a so-called clinical clerk (or, as the British pronounce it, "clark") following sick patients.

Actually, teaching at the bedside was William Osler's great contribution to medical education, first introduced at McGill University and then at the new Johns Hopkins Medical School in Baltimore in 1896.[37] In the nineteenth century, medical teaching was done exclusively in steep walled amphitheatres seating the entire medical school class. In the "pit" was the professor, who, depending on his specialty, would examine, operate on, or deliver the subject patient. This was the closest a medical student ever got to a patient before graduation. On the ward at the bedside, Osler taught his students to reason a problem through, to look for clues when taking a history, to use their powers of observation at physical examination — their eyes, their ears, their sense of touch — and so to link the disease process and the disordered anatomy to the patient's clinical picture in order to arrive at a diagnosis.

In Toronto during the Dirty Thirties, medical education was conducted on a different sort of stage. At all points in a doctor's schooling, those responsible for teaching this Oslerian method were a veritable *dramatis personae*, a colourful and unforgettable cast of characters: they were accomplished, very competent, upright, authoritarian, principled, uncompromising, and unapologetic, and they didn't shrink from applying a little eccentricity and showmanship, using a measure of flair to make a point. They were, for the most part, gentle men and gentlemen. Some were revered and even loved. Some were held in awe but little real affection. A very few were harassing, humiliating bullies and were hated for it. At that time, a far higher premium was placed on one's talent as a teacher than on one's ability to conduct good research, and most professors in Toronto were far better teachers than researchers.

John Charles Boileau Grant, arguably the greatest teacher of anatomy of the twentieth century, came to Toronto in 1930 just in time to teach young George Hendry and his Meds 3T5 classmates. Grant taught students to reason anatomically and not to memorize slavishly. He had the uncanny ability to explain a function or a clinical condition by relating it to some anatomical feature of a bone or a muscle or an organ. He always wore an academic gown when he lectured and invariably began by saying "good morning" to the class. Before the neophyte dissectors approached their assigned cadaver for the first time, Dr. Grant would remind them of the privilege they had been accorded of being able to study human material and that their "natural instincts" would surely lead them "to treat it with the respect due to the dead."[38] This advice is, of course, superfluous today, as it has been many years since medical students learned their anatomy by dissecting cadavers.

W.D. Somerville wrote, "And what a teacher Dr. Grant was! The anatomical drawings he could build up on the blackboard, layer upon layer of coloured chalk, were … unforgettable and he always seemed to be able to tell a story or make some comment which would engrave the subject on your memory."[39]

"His whole bearing as a professor revealed his sense of duty and devotion to his teaching, furtherance of his profession and the pursuit of excellence…. He was an exemplary man."[40]

Some, like dour, unsmiling, monolithic Duncan Graham, the Sir John and Lady Eaton Professor of Medicine, were given shivering respect but little affection. Graham was a great administrator and medical reformer who trained six chairmen of university departments across Canada but who could be "mercilessly harsh with students who made silly statements" or who were slow to pick up his logically based deductive reasoning.[41] He used the Socratic method of teaching, much the same as John Houseman's merciless character Professor Kingsfield in the film *Paper Chase*, and he terrified generations of Toronto medical students with his relentless questioning.

There is a story concerning an unexpected response to "the Prof's" teaching method that would fit quite nicely into a book like Richard Gordon's *Doctor in the House*. During one of his weekly theatre clinics at TGH in the spring of 1939, Duncan Graham was giving a quiet, rather hesitant final-year student a particularly savage roasting when one of this poor lad's classmates, Charles T. ("Robbie") Robertson spoke up in his defence with a sarcastic remark to the professor. After the class, Dr. Graham let Robbie know in unmistakable terms that he was not about to forget this outburst. Two months later, Robbie arrived at TGH for his final oral examination in medicine and was assigned a patient to examine in the solarium at the extreme end of the long Ward I. Robbie completed his examination of the patient and, as was the practice, waited patiently for the first staffman to come along and give him his quiz. He looked down the long corridor and, to his horror, saw Duncan Graham approaching relentlessly closer and closer. Remembering the incident with his classmate, Robbie was appalled at the prospect of having Dr. Graham as his examiner. He saw his medical career coming to an abrupt end. Terrified, he nipped behind the solarium door, froze stock-still, and held his breath. Graham entered the solarium, passed the door, turned, and, with agonizing slowness, walked out of the solarium and up the long ward. Then, as if heaven-sent, appeared Dr. John Hepburn, the senior cardiologist at the TGH and a kinder man than Graham. Robbie emerged from behind the solarium door and pleaded successfully with Hepburn to come and give him his quiz before the professor returned. Happily, Dr. Graham was none the wiser. Robbie passed, and the rest, as they say, is history.[42]

Some teachers could bring a carefully measured showmanship to classroom or conference. Such a man was the superb surgeon Roscoe Graham, always elegantly turned out in a three-piece powder blue suit with flower in buttonhole. He would have a problem case presented to him, of which he had no prior knowledge, in front of an amphitheatre full of senior medical students. He would call for diagnostic suggestions from the assembled students, writing down all twenty or so on the blackboard. Giving his reasons for exclusion, he would then proceed to rub out all but one. On the desk in front of him would be a sealed envelope containing the correct diagnosis. In a performance redolent of the Academy Awards, Graham would tear it open, glance at the contents, and with a magnificent sweep of his hand toss the paper to his adoring audience. He would then depart the room with similar panache. It is hardly necessary to add that he was always correct!

Some were lofty and imperious like Toronto's famed elder statesman of surgery Frederick Newton Gisborne Starr, whose picture hanging in my old fraternity house has him resplendent with AOA key dangling on his watch chain, looking down on the rest of us with his steely gaze, suffering fools poorly.

Some were masters of the written and spoken word like William Boyd, the elegant professor of pathology who (like his brother-in-law, J.C.B.

Grant) came down from the University of Manitoba. He arrived in 1937, too late to have had a part in George Hendry's pre-clinical education. However, their paths may have crossed after Hendry took up his teaching appointment at the TGH in 1939. Boyd achieved his fame with seven textbooks, including his superb *Textbook of Pathology*, beautifully written and replete with vivid metaphors from the classical literature, Greek mythology, and the Bible. Like Osler, Boyd made the intimate links between pathological lesions and the patient's clinical picture the foundation of his writing and his teaching.[43]

There was only one Alan Brown, the legendary and dictatorial professor of paediatrics at the University of Toronto and paediatrician-in-chief at the old Hospital for Sick Children (67 College Street) from 1919 to 1951. There is no question that Alan Brown's heyday at HSC was the ten years of the Great Depression. By 1929, he had established himself as an excellent diagnostician and a strong and unwavering proponent of preventive paediatrics. He managed to convince the equally flamboyant and autocratic Premier Mitchell Hepburn of the much-debated wisdom of making the Dionne quintuplets wards of the Province of Ontario and of the urgent necessity for the pasteurization of milk.

Alan Brown lived with the unshakeable conviction that he was always right. His word was law, and anybody — colleague, intern, nurse, or administrator — who disobeyed his orders or (God forbid) opposed him was fired on the spot. Brown could be harsh and even cruel to parents, particularly the mothers of his small patients. He rode his residents and interns unmercifully; he abused and betrayed his junior staff and senior colleagues. He could make the life of a medical student an undiluted hell, with his scathing sarcasm, humiliation, and bullying. He never could see the error of his ways and he was in fact his own worst enemy. Someone has described his professional life as "a studied career of autocracy," and yet there were always those who would come to this mercurial man's defence.[44]

The stories about Alan Brown are legion but one of the most apt (and reminiscent of Richard Gordon's *Doctor in the House*) concerned an incident that occurred nearly a decade after George Hendry's time during Brown's last year in the old HSC building. It seems that he took to locking his classroom door so that late-coming students would not interrupt his lecture. In January 1950, the "vet" year (consisting of ex-corvette captains, bomber squadron commanders, and battalion colonels) had been locked out once too often, and they retaliated by locking Dr. Brown out. Furious and characteristically oblivious to the point, he roared over to demand extreme penitence of the miscreants. The dean, Joe Macfarlane, had been a brigadier overseas in the war and, less than sympathetic with Brown's badly bruised ego, suggested that he settle the thing calmly with the vets, which Brown did.

W.B. Hendry was cut from different cloth. "The Chief" could stimulate loyalty instinctively by example and not as a requirement. He was a gentle man and a gentleman. Very few physician-professors can claim to have been so truly loved by all: students, house staff, colleagues, and patients.[45]

In those days, medical students were overwhelmingly male, younger than their present-day counterparts, and decidedly single. Nobody could afford marriage. Perhaps they were not as academically brilliant but they probably had more enthusiasm and they definitely had more passion. Medicine was a great adventure. They didn't question experience and took more on faith. Values like duty, honour, and integrity were accepted without negotiation or debate. Sacrifice was expected. They were more respectful of their teachers and were probably more intimidated by them. They didn't take themselves as seriously as today's students. They had more fun and they poked more fun. Using "Daffydil," the annual Meds show, as their ultimate weapon, they could skewer their oppressors. This was the stuff of good stories and they abound.

The curriculum then required much more hands-on learning. The calendar for the Faculty of Medicine mandated that senior medical students "take charge of cases in the wards of the hospital," "attend [obstetrical] patients in their homes," "be certified for at least twelve autopsies," "[master] the principles and art of prescription writing," "[lead] demonstrations to small groups in the use of the fluroscope," and "give at least six anaesthetics before graduation." The student were also required to complete a long list of surgical procedures, including the administration of local anaesthetics, the injection of varicose veins, the passage of duodenal and stomach tubes, the making of incisions, the suturing of wounds, the aspiration of chest and abdomen, the aspiration of joints, the puncture of the spine, and "the passage of catheters and sounds" — but absolutely nothing about contraception, sexuality, or erectile dysfunction![46]

On February 28, 1930, someone took an aerial photograph of the Toronto General Hospital complex bounded by College, Elizabeth, and Gerrard streets and University Avenue, at that time much narrower and leading into a very thin Queen's Park Circle. If one were to take a photo of the same view today, the back of the long, sprawling 1912 hospital building facing College Street and the Banting Institute opposite would be completely obscured by the enormous space-age MARS medical research complex. The spanking new, soon-to-be-opened Private Patients Pavilion, with nine operating suites, six separate labour and delivery rooms, and 321 private rooms with individual beds, faces University Avenue. This "largest and most glittering jewel ... added to this royal crown of buildings." The TGH, giving one the "impression of being within a private hotel of select character," was fortunately completed just after the stock market crash of October 1929 at a cost of $3.8 million.[47]

I can vividly recall my father, a consultant obstetrician at the Toronto General Hospital, parking our car on University Avenue on his way in to make his rounds on a Sunday morning later on in the 1930s. Out of nowhere would appear two or three middle-aged men, each begging to wash the car for a quarter. Like any impatient seven-year-old boy, I would shift from foot to foot in the little ambulance entrance, waiting for him to return, all the time smelling the ether that had seeped into the bricks and fascinated by the teleautograph, an antiquated facsimile machine with mechanical pens that transmitted written messages between various floors and the main switchboard there at the little entrance.[48]

On the southeast corner of College and Elizabeth streets stands that magnificent 1875 pile, the Victoria Hospital for Sick Children, then the fiefdom of Dr. Alan Brown, its legendary paediatrician-in-chief. A new HSC will finally be built in 1952 on the south side of Gerrard Street opposite the Private Patients Pavilion, but for now this lot is occupied by a cluster of old row houses.

The newly completed Banting Institute, housing pathology and research laboratories, will be formally opened on September 16, 1930.[49] The new Women's College Hospital will be built in 1934 at the top of Elizabeth Street north of College Street.

In spite of the number of open (and snow-covered) spaces between buildings in the 1930 photograph, the Toronto General Hospital was the largest private non-government-supported institution of its kind in North America. In the end, however, good medical schools are known less for their bricks and mortar than for their people, and in the 1930s the University of Toronto's Faculty of Medicine was no different.

No records survive that tell of George Hendry's academic progress through medical school, but "Torontonensis," the university yearbook, and the University of Toronto's famous student newspaper, the *Varsity*, abundantly confirm his superb ability as a hockey player, culminating in his captaincy of the U of T Blues Senior OHA team in 1934. There is little doubt that if George had not pursued a career in medicine, he could easily have played with the Toronto Maple Leafs.

Jack Hendry's tragic death in February 1934 was an enormous blow to the family. George felt that he must now concentrate completely on his

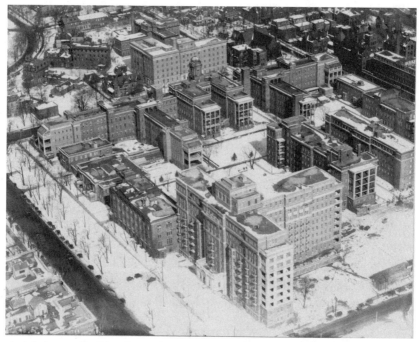

Aerial photograph of brand new Private Patients Pavilion in the lower right corner of the Toronto General Hospital block, taken on February 28, 1930. Note the equally new Banting Institute building (top, on north side of College Street facing the TGH), the Burnside Lying-in Hospital (now replaced by the towering space-age MARS medical research building) facing Elizabeth Street (top right), the then-narrow University Avenue (left), and just a hint of the very narrow Queen's Park Circle (top left). There were many open spaces in 1930 that will be filled by 2006. (Courtesy of Rick Teminski, Northway-Photomap, Inc.)

studies, and so he made the decision to retire from the hockey team during the 1934–35 season, his final year in medical school. Nevertheless, at graduation, he won the Gold Headed Cane,[50] awarded annually to the medical school's finest athlete. Because he had dropped out of hockey, George, in a characteristic gesture, gave the cane to Frank Shipp, his great friend, teammate, and classmate.

At convocation on June 17, 1935, a very proud father, Professor William Belfry Hendry, presented the degree of Doctor of Medicine to his son, George Ainslie Hendry.

Young Dr. Hendry (and he looks very young indeed in his graduation picture) took up his appointment as junior intern at the Toronto General Hospital on July 1, 1935. The internship of old could be a dispiriting and exhausting job. Interns, or "housemen" as they were called, were paid nothing and were provided with their uniforms and board only. They could easily work one hundred hours a week, sometimes more. Constantly at the beck and call of staffmen, residents, and senior nurses, the harried houseman took endless histories and examined unnumbered patients, assisted in the operating room, delivered babies at all hours, attended in

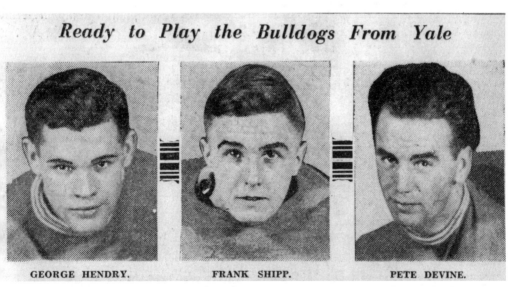

"Ready to Play the Bulldogs From Yale": U of T Senior OHA hockey teammates Hendry, Shipp, Devine. (Toronto Globe and Mail, December 16, 1934.)

the emergency department, and did all manner of routine laboratory work during nights and weekends, because in those days that wasn't in the lab technicians' job description. Unless you had independent means, marriage was out of the question.

It would not be an exaggeration to say that an internship in those days was a form of indentured servitude and continued to be so until a decade or more after the Second World War. Nobody complained; nobody dared. It was all rather like a continuing fraternity initiation that was expected and accepted without demur. Some staffmen (once again, there were no women until much later) were demanding workaholics, some were mean, and some were openly eccentric. Not all newly graduated physicians did an internship, but if you wanted to be a specialist or, better still, a teacher, there was no other way. You had to endure the refiner's fire without a murmur.

Still, it wasn't all bad. You could overlook an awful lot if your staffman was a good mentor, and many of the staff of Toronto's teaching hospitals were very good indeed. Life as an intern could be quite bearable as long as you could have a little fun from time to time. Stories abound of almost Munchausian pranks from that time. Young, baby-faced interns would grow mustaches to bolster their confidence and enhance their professional mien.

Postgraduate training after the internship was shorter and less well organized in 1936 than it would become after the Second World War. George Hendry did two years as a "senior houseman" (resident) in obstetrics and gynaecology at the Toronto General Hospital and then

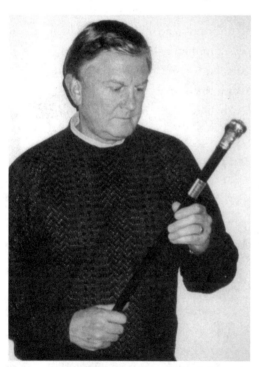

Frank Shipp's eldest son, Peter, holding the Gold Headed Cane, emblematic of one of the highest honours in university athletics. The cane had been awarded to George Hendry, who immediately presented it to Frank, saying he was more deserving of the honour. (Courtesy of Peter Shipp.)

decided to take an additional year as a senior houseman in general surgery at St. Michael's Hospital in Toronto. This was a sensible move because taking a similar position at the TGH would mean competing with surgical residents there for less practical operative experience, and St. Michael's had some excellent senior surgeons. In any event, he was the professor's son, and the move out of the TGH, if only for a year, was prudent politically. Four years later, there were four days on board the destroyer HMCS *Ottawa* when George Hendry probably gave silent thanks for experience gained there.

George Hendry finished his year in general surgery at St. Michael's on June 30, 1939. His formal postgraduate training as an obstetrician and gynaecologist complete, he was given a junior staff appointment in the Department of Obstetrics and

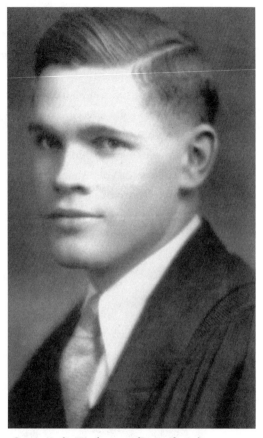

George Ainslie Hendry at graduation from the University of Toronto Faculty of Medicine in June 1935, age twenty-four. (Courtesy of Carol Hendry Duffus.)

Gynaecology at the Toronto General Hospital and an appointment as teaching fellow in the University of Toronto Medical School. He went into practice with my father, James C. Goodwin, at 516 Medical Arts Building, which had also been his late father's office. He moved out of the family home at 286 Russell Hill Road and leased a house at 339 Walmer Road just north of Casa Loma.

In the spring of 1939, Their Majesties King George VI and Queen Elizabeth made their famous Royal Tour of Canada, the first time in history that a reigning British monarch had set foot on an overseas dominion. This carefully orchestrated visit was made for two vital reasons. Firstly, the

British government was fully aware of the imminence of war, even if the public at home and overseas was not, and the royal visit was intended to have enormous inspirational value in rallying the Empire to the colours. Secondly, citizens of the Empire, more so than the public at home in Britain, were still reeling from the unprecedented Abdication Crisis of 1936 and its damaging effect on the stability of the monarchy.

The tour proved to be a huge success,[51] but the prospect of war was not uppermost in the minds of the Canadian people. The Great Depression dragged on, and many were still on the dole. The First World War (which everyone referred to as the Great War) had come to an unsatisfactory conclusion a little over twenty years before with an armistice rather than an unconditional surrender. Its veterans, not all that old, paraded every Labour Day in the 1930s at the Canadian National Exhibition in Toronto. The CNE brass even managed to trot out a few surviving Boer War (1899–1902) veterans! We knew about the Nazi takeover of Austria, and about the Munich sellout of Czechoslovakia, but another war? Unthinkable! We were lulled by British Prime Minister Neville Chamberlain's words on September 27, 1938: "How horrible, fantastic, incredible it is that we should be digging trenches and trying on gas-masks here because of a quarrel in a far-away country between people of whom we know nothing."[52] The truly horrible thing was that the "far-away country" he was referring to was Czechoslovakia, not Outer Mongolia, and just three days later Mr. Chamberlain was to sell out that country to Adolf Hitler at Munich.

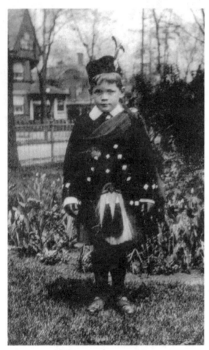

George Hendry, age nine, in highland garb outside 154 Walmer Road, Toronto, in 1920. This was one of two such suits given to the Goodwin boys when the Hendry boys had outgrown them. (Courtesy of Carol Hendry Duffus.)

We did indeed go to war in early September 1939, and until May 1940 the conflict was so utterly

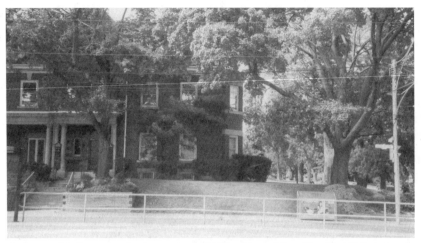

As she passed by in an open landau carriage with King George VI on May 22, 1939, during the royal visit to Canada, Queen Elizabeth waved at the two Goodwin boys dressed in the Hendry highlander suits standing on this terraced lawn in front of the Hendry home on St. Clair Avenue at Russell Hill Road, Toronto. (Courtesy of Dr. James Goodwin.)

unlike the stygian horrors of 1914–18 that it was soon dubbed the "Phony War." George Hendry was doubtless the sort of fellow who would get right down to the nearest recruiting office and join up. There was ample family tradition: his father had been decorated for distinguished service in the First World War and his brother had served in the peacetime militia. But his father and brother were gone now, and the sole surviving male in the family should see after his mother's welfare. His postgraduate training was finished and he was clearly anxious to begin practice. True, some of his contemporaries had joined up, including his best friend, Frank Shipp, but Canadians did seem rather nonchalant about the war at that point.

As well as his new staff position at the Toronto General Hospital, George had an appointment as a consultant in obstetrics and gynaecology at the Women's College Hospital just across from the Toronto General and at the north end of Elizabeth Street. It was here, one day in May 1940, while he was making his rounds, that he read a note on his patient's chart written by a young nurse that described an enema as having produced "wonderful results." He could barely suppress a laugh. Thus he became aware of twenty-one-year-old Elizabeth Audrie Summers, who had just graduated from the School of Nursing at Women's College Hospital. Betty Summers (she was forever "Betty" to her family and her many friends) was

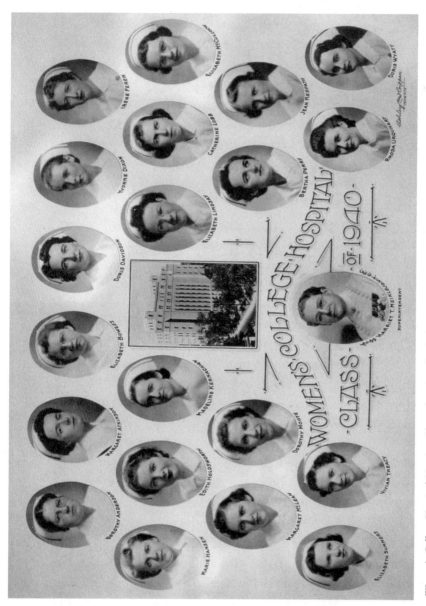

Women's College Hospital Nursing Class of 1940. Elizabeth Summers is in the lower left of the photograph. (Courtesy of Women's College Hospital Archives.)

born in her grandparents' home in London, Ontario, on September 11, 1918, exactly two months before the Armistice ended the First World War. Her grandfather had predicted that there would be fireworks that evening, and sure enough (as her daughters proclaimed in their eulogy at her funeral) "Betty Summers came into this world with a luminous sparkle which she would carry with her always."

Her father was a skilled jeweller, and when, a few years later, a better position beckoned in Toronto, the family moved there. Betty spent summer vacations at a Girl Guide camp on Lake Couchiching and later on the Muskoka Lakes. There in Northern Ontario, she developed an abiding love for nature, birds, and Indian lore. She passed this gift on to her family in 1951 when she purchased a summer home in Burks Falls, Ontario. During her high school years at Parkdale Collegiate Betty determined to train as a nurse. Instead of taking the conventional route and enrolling in one of the major teaching hospitals like the Toronto General, she decided to enter the training program at Women's College, which had just moved from its old site on Rushholme Road into a new building three yeas before.

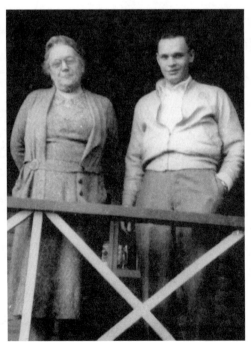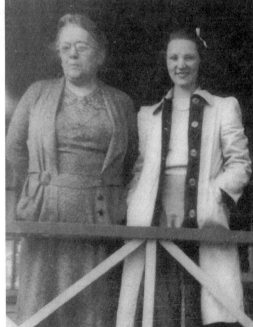

Left: George and his mother at the Bala cottage, fall 1940. Right: George's mother and Betty Summers, on the porch at Bala, fall 1940. (Courtesy of Betty Summers Minogue.)

In those days, young, single doctors just starting out as a university consultant (George was now twenty-nine) and young, newly graduated student nurses (Betty was twenty-one) had to be pretty circumspect about beginning a relationship. Toronto society, and especially that centred around the health professions, was particularly vigilant about any breach of propriety. However, nothing daunted, they did begin a relationship and they soon fell in love. One gruff but kindly nursing supervisor at Women's College would look the other way while Betty slipped out so that George could take her across to afternoon tea in the Round Room of the ten-year-old Eaton's College Street store. He took her to dances, out to dinner with old friends, and, of course, he took her home to mother. They were indeed an item: they weren't formally engaged but they had a very considerable understanding.

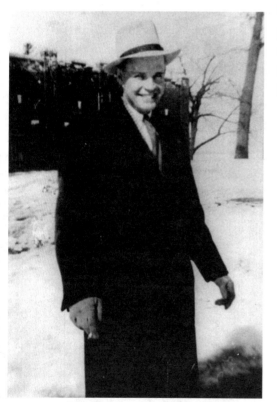

George told Betty that he would be giving her his mother's engagement ring. In the popular expression of the day, the world was truly George Hendry's oyster.

The new consultant: a smiling George Hendry outside the "Burnside" at the Toronto General Hospital with fedora, gloves, and cigarette, December 1940. (Courtesy of Betty Summers Minogue.)

"Is Anxious to Have His Entry Hastened" 3

*M*y father, James C. Goodwin, died suddenly on August 3, 1953. That summer, between my second and third medical year at the University of Toronto, I was an officer cadet in the Royal Canadian Air Force working in physiological research at the Institute of Aviation Medicine in Toronto. When I returned to work a few days later, I was called to the office of IAM's commanding officer, Wing Commander Hugh J. Bright, a 1936 graduate in medicine at the university and a good friend to George Hendry. He offered his condolences and then told me the following story.

After he had finished his postgraduate training and had joined my father in private obstetrical practice in Toronto, George Hendry fell in love with a wonderful girl and they were just about to become engaged. But, Bright told me, at some point George went alone to a party, had too much to drink, and took another girl (a nurse) to bed, with pregnancy the result. George felt he had to do the honourable thing: he had to call off his engagement and marry the other woman. Then it turned out that there was no pregnancy; she had made the whole thing up to entrap George. Hugh Bright gave no names and no dates. He said he was angry with George for making a stupid mistake, as only a very good friend would be. He told me that George joined the navy to get as far away from Toronto as he could. He said that George was heartbroken and that much of the life went out of him after that.

Hugh Bright made this stunning disclosure fifty-three years ago, but it is etched in my memory. I was grieving for my father and I must have decided not to speak about this to anybody, not even to my mother.

It added an unforeseen and startling new dimension to the story of George Hendry's heroism and death that I had been brought up with.

I was totally immersed in my medical studies and then my professional career, so it was years before I could begin to set this story down. By the time I did, nearly all the people — those who knew and loved George, in Toronto and on board the *Ottawa* — were dead. The testimony of seven women in their eighties, Carol Hendry Duffus, Betty Summers Minogue, and five survivors of the Toronto General Hospital nursing class of 1938, plus a couple of legal documents and four letters are all that remain today to fill in the blanks in the story. How many times have I wished that I could raise some ghosts!

Although only fragments of this story survive, this much is true: For some inexplicable reason, George went alone to a party at or very near the Toronto General Hospital, probably sometime in January 1941. Jean Matthews, a nurse working at the Burnside Hospital, apparently attended this gathering as well. George had too much to drink, and on this particular night, there can be no doubt that he was in bed with Jean Matthews.

In those days, doctors were exquisitely careful about taking a

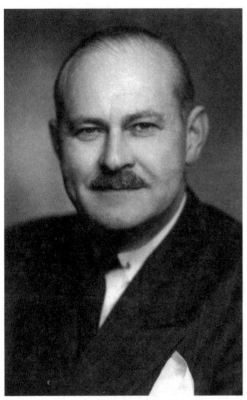

James C. ("Jimmie") Goodwin, MA, MD, 1902–53. W.B. Hendry's assistant, then colleague, and finally cherished friend. George Ainslie Hendry's good friend and partner in practice. My father. (Courtesy of Dr. James Goodwin.)

social drink or exposing themselves to even a hint of sexual misconduct, particularly young doctors with teaching appointments at prestigious institutions like the Toronto General Hospital and the University of Toronto's medical school. This sort of caution would apply most particularly to a young doctor who was the scion of a medical family like the Hendrys. Added to these strictures was George Hendry's later admission that he had an almost toxic vulnerability to alcohol. So it is astonishing that he would let down his guard and take such a ruinous risk.

Jean Isobel Matthews entered the first year of her nursing education at the Toronto General Hospital on September 25, 1935. One of her surviving classmates, Mildred Hall, said she was a "pretty, petite redhead" who came from Vancouver, British Columbia. At age twenty-eight (born June 3, 1907, in Halifax, Nova Scotia), she was a good ten years older than the average member of her nursing class. It was well known that Jean came from the moneyed class, while most of her classmates couldn't rub two cents together. She was a member of a distinguished, well-to-do Canadian family. Her father, Alfred Joseph Matthews, had been killed in action in Flanders on February 26, 1916. Her widowed mother lived in comfort in Vancouver. One of her father's brothers, Robert Charles Matthews, had been minister of national revenue in R.B. Bennett's government in 1933. Another, Albert Edward Matthews, was lieutenant-governor of Ontario

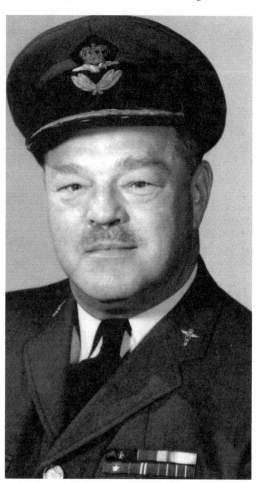

Wing commander Hugh J. Bright, MD, as commanding officer, Institute of Medicine, Toronto, in 1953. A good friend of George and Betty's, Hugh told me the other side of this tragic story on August 10, 1953, one week after my father died. (Courtesy of H.J. Bright, Jr., MD.)

when his niece was in Nursing School at the Toronto General Hospital and had presented the diplomas at her graduation. Jean Matthews must have thought of herself as George Hendry's social equal.

Jean was not a treacherous person, but she was undoubtedly desperate. She was four years older than George; she was far older than her nursing classmates. She probably felt that she was in danger of becoming a spinster. She must have thought she had a chance with George and, accordingly, took advantage of the situation.

Some of the details of this tragic encounter are based on speculation and rumour, much of it critical of Jean. George was the beau ideal: everybody admired this guy. He had been a great university athlete; he was by all accounts an excellent surgeon with a very promising future; he was kind and always helpful to house staff and nursing students, quiet and unassuming, and undeniably attractive. He was all but engaged to Betty Summers and it's unlikely that he could have known Jean Matthews in anything but a completely professional relationship before that evening. It is, however, indisputable that he had just made the worst mistake of his life.

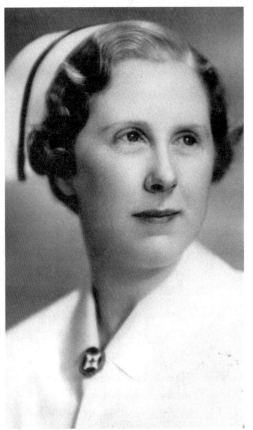

Graduation photograph of Jean Isobel Matthews, Toronto General Hospital Nursing Class of 1938. (Courtesy of Margaret Frazier.)

Jean Matthews probably became infatuated with George Hendry while working with him at the Burnside Hospital. When she ran into him at this party, she may well have decided to make the most of the opportunity. What appears at first blush to have been a premeditated seduction may have started out as an artless fling that got out of hand. It's hardly surprising that George's cousin, Carol Hendry

Duffus, and his sweetheart, Betty Summers Minogue, are convinced otherwise. They feel that Jean trapped George and seduced him.

George told not a soul about any of this until, in the last week of March, Jean told him that she was pregnant. Why did he not confide in Betty soon after this disaster? Probably he was hoping against hope that nothing unfortunate had happened and that the whole thing would just blow over.

A woman usually needs to miss at least two menstrual periods (referred to as *amenorrhoea*) and to experience telltale symptoms such as nausea and breast tenderness for her to be suspicious of early pregnancy. Jean Matthews was a graduate nurse and would have reported this possibility to George Hendry sooner rather than later. So an interval of eight to ten weeks between their encounter sometime in January and Jean's disclosure in late March would be about right. Whether she was amenorrhoeic or not really doesn't matter. The critical fact is that she told George she was pregnant and he believed her.

George had now made not one but two appalling errors of judgement. He'd gone alone to this hospital party; Jean Matthews was pregnant and he was responsible. It seems that he decided to trust Jean's story and do nothing at all to confirm the pregnancy for himself. He balked at having anybody else examine Jean, fearing that the secret would get around the hospital, and he certainly didn't examine her himself. Betty Summers Minogue told me in 2005, "It's a haunting thought to this day. I'm sure [George] wanted to keep this disgusting news quiet. Thinking back, he was too trusting and did not want to be ridiculed by his friends, especially your father [James C. Goodwin]." Clearly, George felt it was his duty to marry Jean and to sacrifice his happiness with Betty Summers.

George Hendry was acutely aware of the effect that a scandal would have on his family, especially on his mother, who in the last seven years had lost her husband and her other son. George was also aware that the Toronto General Hospital had to be protected from any taint of wrongdoing or immoral behaviour. Particularly during the thirties and forties, the hospital was the flagship teaching institution of the University of Toronto's medical school. It was lofty and unassailable. To generations of irreverent medical students, it was known as the "House of Lords." All the leading professors, teachers, and heads of the university's clinical departments were on its staff. George's father, W.B. Hendry, had been the hospital's obstetrician and gynaecologist-in-chief. An added embarrassment was the fact that Jean Matthews's uncle was Ontario's lieutenant-governor.

To understand how a man could be duped and entrapped into marriage during the Dirty Thirties and beyond, one must be aware how strongly upper-crust Toronto society felt about duty, sacrifice, morality, and the sanctity of marriage. The rules of moral conduct were inviolable. Premarital sex was anathema. A single gentleman treated a single lady with honour, and if through some careless indiscretion she became pregnant, there was but one course of action open to him. It was his duty to marry her. This was not debatable and certainly not negotiable. Ugly scandals threatening a family's reputation were skillfully squelched and the necessary ceremony performed quietly and without delay.

Divorce was almost impossible to obtain. Contraception was primitive and extremely unreliable. The subject was rigorously omitted in the medical school curriculum. Sexually transmitted infections were called "venereal diseases": they could be crippling, and the available medical treatment for them was crude and ineffective. Abortion was a back alley crime and was frequently fatal. Single girls would go away to homes to have their babies and were obliged to put them up for adoption. The only single parents were widows, and couples never lived openly together "without benefit of clergy."

George had undoubtedly not forgotten that in 1932, when he was partway through medical school, the most celebrated Canadian of that time, Dr. (later Sir) Frederick Banting, he of insulin fame, was publicly involved in a very messy divorce case. And then there was the ultimately public scandal of the Abdication Crisis of 1936, with King Edward VIII choosing the twice-divorced Wallis Warfield Simpson over his duty as monarch. In a stern and unforgiving letter written in July 1938, nineteen months after his abdication, Queen Mary rebuked her son, the Duke of Windsor (formerly King Edward VIII), for shirking his royal duty: "I do not think that you have ever realised the shock, which the attitude you took up caused your family and the whole nation. It seemed inconceivable to those who had made such sacrifices during the war [the Great War] that you, as their King, refused a lesser sacrifice."[53]

One night soon after Jean's disclosure, as George was driving Betty home after her shift at Women's College Hospital, he told her quietly that he couldn't marry her "right now." He told her that Jean Matthews was pregnant by him and that he was going to have to marry her.[54] He tried to soften the blow by promising her that this was certainly not going to be a permanent contract. Betty tried to make light of it by telling him, "That's OK, I've made other plans next week, anyway." Early on the morning of April 3, 1941, as she was riding home in a streetcar after a night on duty at Women's College, she saw George and Jean passing through the iron gates outside Jean's apartment building at 219 College Street on their way out of town.

Jean Isobel Matthews and Dr. George Ainslie Hendry were married quickly and quietly on April 3, 1941, in Preston (now Cambridge), Ontario. The ceremony was performed by a United Church minister, the Reverend E. Milton Morrow, whose wife obligingly acted as one of the witnesses. It was a wedding in name only: the customary members of a wedding party were conspicuously absent. Other than the need for secrecy and haste, the reason for selecting Preston is unknown. There was no celebration and certainly no wedding trip. On their return to Toronto, the couple moved into the rented house at 339 Walmer Road. They slept in separate beds and George never touched Jean intimately again. On April 9, 1941, a very terse announcement of the marriage was inserted by Jean's mother (far away in British Columbia) in the *Globe and Mail*: "Hendry-Matthews — Mrs. A.J. Matthews, Vancouver, announces the marriage of her daughter, Jean Isobel, to Dr. George Ainslie Hendry, Toronto, the son of Mrs. W.B. Hendry and the late Dr. Hendry, Toronto."

That was all. There was none of the customary flowery description of the bride's dress and her going away attire or the usual cataloguing of the wedding party. Most people around the TGH heard about it as a very hush-hush happening and all were taken completely by surprise.

It could only have been a day or two after this furtive marriage ceremony that Jean told George that she wasn't pregnant after all. She may have skipped a couple of periods, which can mimic early pregnancy, or she may have had no suggestive symptoms at all. In the end, this sort of speculation is irrelevant. The salient fact is that there was no pregnancy and Jean kept this fact from George until after he had married her.

Jean's TGH nursing classmates were stunned by the news. Bernice Scott spoke for them: "Jean told George she was pregnant but then turned out not to be. We couldn't believe that any of us could do such a thing." Another classmate, Sally Eede Hillier, had heard that George told Jean, "I'll marry you, but I'll never live with you." She was overseas with the 15th Canadian General Hospital in 1942 when she heard that George had made it to a float when the ship was sunk, but then (some felt that) he was so depressed that he just let himself go and was lost.

George's old friend, the late Arthur Squires, could confirm every detail of this sad story, as could both Carol Hendry Duffus and the late Betty Summers Minogue. Carol Hendry Duffus continues to be very bitter about the manner in which Jean Matthews deceived George. In a letter to Betty Summers on September 26, 1942, thirteen days after George had died at sea, Elizabeth Hendry wrote, "I know how you both were cheated out of your happiness."

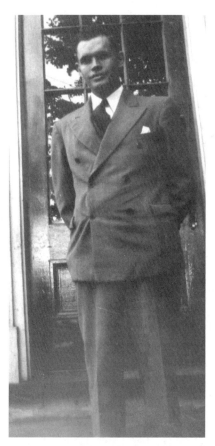

G.A. Hendry, MD, at the front door of 339 Walmer Road, Toronto, in April 1941. (Courtesy of Margaret Frazier.)

There might be a strong temptation to denounce Jean Matthews, but there is more to pity here than there is to condemn. There is no doubt at all that Jean loved George Hendry, but she was willing to break all the rules in order to snag him. Although extremely unlikely, it is conceivable that George might have had sexual liaisons with other women before this. It could even be argued that he might have had a relationship with Jean Matthews before this. None of this, however, can free Jean Matthews from the charge that she concealed a fictitious pregnancy until she was safely married to him.

In photographs taken of George Hendry before and after his humiliating deception, there is an obvious change. This is not the same man.

Before this disaster, he's outgoing, confident, happy, and smiling. After, he's glum, indifferent, sullen, or frankly sheepish. In one snapshot with Jean, he looks almost bloated. There would be no more smiles for the camera.

Throughout this devastating episode, George was at once embarrassed, naïve, far too trusting and gullible, angry, ashamed, and humiliated. Betty Summers Minogue says, "He was all of these things, but he always kept his feelings to himself."

He shunned Jean. He couldn't abandon her, but they slept in separate beds from then on. The fatal mistake in January was the only intimacy Jean ever had with George Hendry. It was never repeated.

George was now determined to go to war as quickly as possible. For obvious reasons, he was intent upon getting as far away as possible from Toronto and from Jean. This probably dictated his desire to join the navy, with an East Coast posting firmly in mind.

In a memorandum dated April 12, 1941 (nine days after the wedding), to Captain J.O. Cossette, RCN,[55] the naval secretary at the Department of National Defence in Ottawa, S.P. Wheelock, the private secretary to the minister of national defence for naval services, wrote, "I am advised that Dr. George Hendry, of Toronto, who is on call for the RCNVR, is anxious to have his entry hastened and would like to be included in the next draft of medical doctors, if it is possible so to do." George didn't have long to wait.

On April 18, 1941, he received a letter from Naval Secretary Cossette that stated in part, "Should you wish to have your name placed on the roster for consideration when vacancies arise in the Naval Medical Service, you should interview the Commanding Officer of the Toronto Division RCNVR, at 165 Lakeshore Boulevard."

Then on May 8, 1941, the naval secretary sent the following memorandum to the commanding officer of the Toronto Division RCNVR and the commanding officer of the Atlantic Coast at HMC Dockyard, Halifax: "Dr. George A. Hendry, of 516 Medical Arts Building, Toronto has offered his services as Surgeon Lieutenant RCNVR (Temp). If medically fit and in your opinion suitable for entry as an officer, he is to be entered as a Surgeon Lieutenant RCNVR (Temp) and drafted to Halifax as soon as he can wind up his private affairs."

There is a very formal document in which the minister of national defence of the Dominion of Canada appoints him "Surgeon Lieutenant RCNVR (Temporary) to HMCS [His Majesty's Canadian Ship] *Stadacona* [Naval Headquarters ashore in Halifax and the site of HMC Dockyard], the appointment to take effect in Halifax on 23 May 1941."

George now took steps to begin divorce proceedings. As the Hendry family lawyer did not practise family and divorce law, the case was referred to an eminent Toronto lawyer who did, Mr. W.W. McLaughlin, senior partner of the firm McLaughlin, Johnston, Moorhead and MacAulay.

George made a will dated May 21, 1941, the day before he left for Halifax to join the navy. (See Appendix A.) The executors were "my mother, Elizabeth Robertson Hendry and my friend, Dr. James C. Goodwin." His mother had been well provided for, and so George left half his estate "to my aunt, Miss Mary Diana Hendry" (his aunt Mame), one-quarter "to my wife, Jean Isobel Hendry," and one-quarter "to Miss Elizabeth Audrey Summers." The will was also handled by Mr. W.W. McLaughlin.

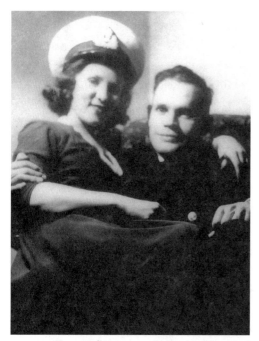

George in his new naval officer's uniform and Betty sporting his new cap at Hugh Bright's apartment on the evening of May 21, 1941. George left on the train for Halifax the next day. Betty would never see him again. (Courtesy of Betty Summers Minogue.)

While Jean languished at home alone on Walmer Road, George and Betty were invited to Hugh and Gertrude Bright's apartment to babysit the Brights' infant daughter so they could be together in those last few evenings before he left for Halifax and the navy.

On May 21, the night before George left on the overnight train for Halifax, he and Betty said goodbye for the last time at Hugh and Gertrude Bright's apartment. She never saw him again. An old photograph shows a sad George in his brand new uniform with Betty on his lap, wearing his new officer's cap at a jaunty angle. The next day, before he went down to Union Station for the Halifax train, there's a different George looking glum and rather wooden, and Jean, in furs, attempting to put the best face on a very unpromising situation. On arrival in Halifax the next day, he reported for duty and was assigned temporary accommodation in an apartment building at 5244 South Street that went by the rather formidable name of the Alexandra Barracks.

A day or so later, Jean suddenly showed up on the train from Toronto. George was furious. Why didn't he just send her back to Toronto on the next train? Perhaps he didn't want to exacerbate an already humiliating situation back home and so felt obliged to keep her with him. Also, as Jean

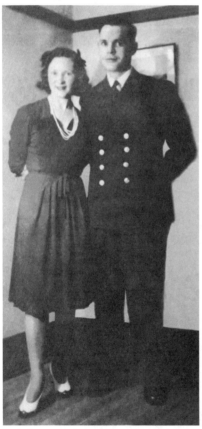 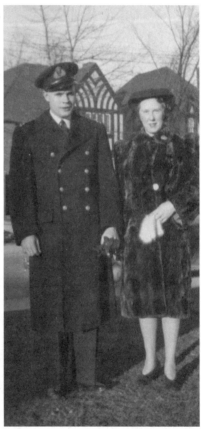

Left: George and Betty at Hugh Bright's apartment, May 21, 1941. (Courtesy of Betty Summers Minogue.)

Right: George looking decidedly glum in his new naval uniform and Jean in furs trying to put on a happy face. Probably taken at 339 Walmer Road, Toronto, on May 22, 1941, the day he left for Halifax. Twenty-four hours after George arrived there, Jean suddenly turned up unannounced. (Courtesy of Margaret Frazier.)

had been born in Halifax and might still have had relatives there, George may have been wary of stirring up family resentment if he abandoned her. There was even a rumour being circulated that she had threatened him with exposure if he were to cast her adrift.

After the standard orientation to the RCN and related training at *Stadacona*, George was posted to the shore establishment HMCS *Protector* in Sydney, Nova Scotia, on August 4, 1941, for more advanced training and medical duties at the RCN Hospital there.

In an intimate letter to Betty on August 26–27 from "RCN Barracks, Sydney," George wrote (cautiously), "I know my letters are very short but that's because I'm afraid someone might peek at them when they're lying around … and we have so many interruptions…. It's hard to complete them at one sitting."

Not surprisingly, he was lonely, too: "I must say though, my own little Darling, that once I have you with me, I'll never be homesick again, only when we're separated, if ever."

He wrote, "I was glad to hear you saw mother. I think she's finally decided to leave on the 2nd [September[56]]. It will take her about five days and how I wish she would bring you along. That would be perfect, Darling,

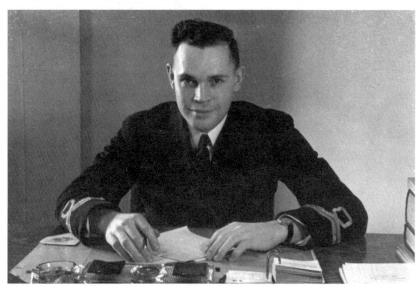

The new surgeon lieutenant at his desk in the RCN hospital at HMCS Protector, *Sydney, Nova Scotia, 1941. (Courtesy of Carol Hendry Duffus.)*

but we can't have everything or even very much at the present time."

Accommodation for married naval officers in Nova Scotia was pretty thin in wartime, but George apparently managed to get into a bungalow. He continued to live apart from Jean:

> As far as our bungalow goes, I think I'll have the chester-field permanently — I might just as well and the months are passing slowly but surely. Just think, Darling, it will soon be September the 3rd, five months since the fatal event.[57] Less than 4 months I hope, Darling, before I return — once the original hearing [for the divorce petition] is over, we can rest assured of the future. What would you think of that? … I do wish we were together now and could have been right along. Never mind though, Darling, the time is coming and nothing can keep us apart soon.

Clearly referring to his intolerance for alcohol, George tells Betty, "Two days ago, two of the officers had birthdays, so the drinks were on

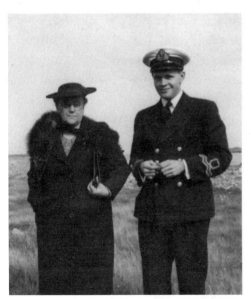 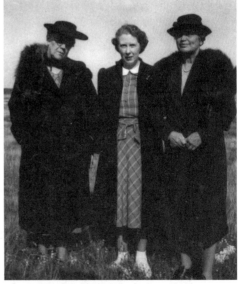

Left: George and his mother in her Buster Keaton hat and foxtail wrap in Sydney, Nova Scotia, September 1941. Right: Elizabeth Hendry, Jean Matthews Hendry, and Mary Diana Hendry on the same beach at Sydney, September 1941. Nobody is smiling. (Courtesy of Carol Hendry Duffus.)

them. Yesterday, another officer had a baby, so the drinks were on him.… And I, Sweetheart, had nothing but Coca-Cola."

George's mother and his aunt Mame did indeed make the long drive to Nova Scotia in early September. There are two photographs taken during that visit at a typical windswept Cape Breton beach. One is of a rather sad looking George Hendry in uniform standing with his mother, who is turned out in fox fur wrap and flat Buster Keaton hat. The other has Jean Matthews Hendry standing between Aunt Mame and George's mother. Nobody is smiling.

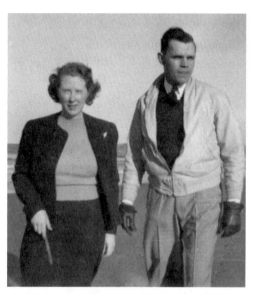

Jean and George on the beach at Sydney, Nova Scotia, September 1941. Jean is attempting to put on a good face for the photo. George is not. (Courtesy of Margaret Frazier.)

Whatever responsibility George felt for taking Jean with him to Sydney after she turned up in Halifax unexpectedly in May, that obligation now seemed to be discharged. Any fleeting hope in Jean's mind that the marriage could be salvaged had certainly flickered and died.

In a letter to my father dated November 23, 1941, George makes reference to preparations for the divorce hearing (see Appendix C):

> I expect to be home on leave soon — arriving on the evening of the 15th of Dec. and leaving again a day or so after Christmas. The other party [his wife, Jean] is going to Ottawa for a while and will arrive in Toronto about the 22nd. That will give me a few days at any rate. I can see Mr. McLaughlin[58] and find out about and establish a spot of evidence before she arrives — I hope. There is a rumour to the effect that a new M.O. is coming to Sydney and that I am due to be drafted. I don't know where or when, but if I get any definite news, I'll try and leave here earlier.

At some point in the fall of 1941, the civilian doctors in Sydney became aware of the fact that there was a young naval surgeon on staff at the RCN Hospital who was a fully trained obstetrician-gynaecologist from Toronto. With only a couple of days' notice, Dr. Fraser Macaulay,[59] a respected senior physician in Sydney, invited George to give a talk on common obstetrical problems to the membership of the Cape Breton Medical Society. These men would have been country general practitioners who delivered most of their pregnant patients in the home. If they had to confine the woman in hospital, they did so using unsophisticated anaesthesia and crude blood transfusion technology. In a very practical talk, George went over the considerable risks that a pregnant woman had to face outside university centres, with forceps and version operations, total breech extraction, the extreme danger of contemporary caesarean section, and the maternal mortality that attended cases of placenta praevia, placental abruption, and eclampsia. In closing, George admitted to his audience, "My own experience [with delivery] in the home is very limited, and ... I hope it will remain so."[60]

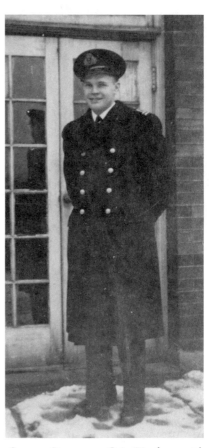

On Sunday, December 7, 1941, Japan suddenly attacked Pearl Harbor. George's Toronto leave and the planned divorce hearing had to be indefinitely postponed. Because she was frantic about the possibility of a Japanese invasion of British Columbia, Jean's mother had moved into a house in Calgary, and Jean joined her there after visiting relatives in Ottawa and Toronto. On

Surgeon Lieutenant G.A. Hendry outside RCN Hospital, Sydney, Nova Scotia, in January 1942, one month before being appointed to HMCS Ottawa. (Courtesy of Carol Hendry Duffus.)

her way through Toronto, Jean called Betty Summers and asked if the two of them could meet. Betty declined, saying that she really didn't think this would accomplish anything. Then Jean said, "I know that George loved you. I know he didn't love me."[61]

His initial naval training complete, Surgeon Lieutenant George Hendry was posted to RCN Barracks at HMCS *Stadacona* on February 20, 1942, in preparation for his posting to sea duty.

HMCS Ottawa *(H 60):*

The Ship and the Ship's Company

*O*n the evening of November 2, 1941, Sub-Lieutenant Latham B. Jenson, RCN (known since his teenage years as "Yogi"), boarded the car ferry SS *Caribou*[62] in North Sydney, Nova Scotia, for the overnight voyage to Port-aux-Basques, Newfoundland, en route to take up his appointment to HMCS *Ottawa* at St. John's. It is no exaggeration to say that for a twenty-year-old, Yogi Jenson had had an eventful (indeed, impressive) naval career.

As a youngster in landlocked Calgary, Yogi had become captivated by the idea of a naval career.[63] The Royal Canadian Naval College in Halifax had been closed in 1922 due to government fiscal stringencies and would not reappear until 1942 as "Royal Roads." So he was obliged to take his schooling as a professional naval officer overseas in England with the Royal Navy. He set off on this grand adventure in August 1938, boarding the transcontinental train in Calgary, "bound for Ottawa and eventually England, the 'Old Country', as my people called it," sailing from Quebec on RMS *Ascania*. During those first three weeks in London before young Jenson joined his first training ship, HMS *Erebus*, in Portsmouth, he was measured for his new uniforms at Gieves, the renowned military tailors, and he called on his uncle, Cedric Naylor, a retired Royal Navy captain with a distinguished record of service in the First World War.[64]

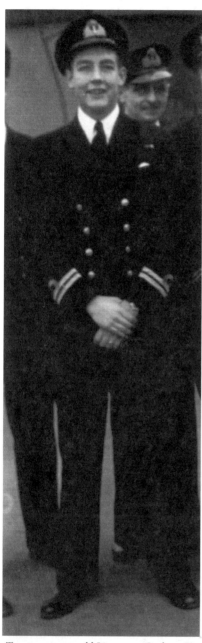

Twenty-two-year-old Lieutenant Latham B. ("Yogi") Jenson in February 1944 when he was first lieutenant of HMCS Algonquin. *(Courtesy of L.B. Jenson.)*

Erebus was a type of ship called a monitor, a sort of floating battery with two enormous fifteen-inch guns. She was moored in Portsmouth Harbour off Whale Island at HMS *Excellent*, the Royal Navy Gunnery School.

There, from dawn to dusk for the next three months, fledgling cadet L.B. Jenson ate, slept, swam, sailed cutters without a rudder, drilled, climbed the tallest mast in the British Empire, and learned navigation, engineering, gunnery, torpedo and signalling, ballroom dancing with fellow cadets (an essential grace for RN officers), and "holystoning" — the repeated polishing of decks with sand applied with sandstone and much elbow grease. Yogi's training continued in this vein until July 1939 on board two old RN cruisers, HMS *Frobisher* and HMS *Vindictive*, when he graduated as midshipman RN and, on September 1, 1939, was appointed to the battle cruiser HMS *Renown*. The ship spent the next weeks "working up" in the Fleet Anchorage at Scapa Flow. She was then ordered to sail for Sierra Leone in West Africa, around the Cape of Good Hope into the Indian Ocean, and back into the South Atlantic in a futile chase of the German "pocket battleship" *Admiral Graf Spee*. She was fuelling in Rio de Janeiro just about the time that the famous raider had scuttled herself on December 17 after the Battle of the River Plate.

Then in April 1940, during the German invasion of Norway, *Renown* was involved in a running gun battle in the Norwegian Sea (the first big ship engagement since the naval battle of Jutland in 1916) with the battle cruisers *Scharnhorst* and *Gneisenau*, damaging the latter seriously in the process. The only damage to *Renown* was a single shot to her stern that destroyed the midshipmen's quarters and obliterated Yogi's journal with its collection of ship drawings. The day before this set-to (April 8), one of *Renown's* escorting destroyers, *Glowworm*, lost a man overboard and turned back to search for him. She suddenly ran into the German heavy cruiser *Admiral Hipper* and, in an unequal contest, rammed her adversary and then sank with heavy loss of life.[65]

From July to December 1940, Midshipman L.B. Jenson, RCN, was appointed to the Tribal class destroyer HMS *Matabele* to put in what was called "small ship time," a major element of a naval officer's training. His captain was the aloof and patrician Commander Robert St. Vincent Sherbrooke, who later won the Victoria Cross when he commanded the destroyer HMS *Onslow* in a ferocious gun battle in the Barents Sea in December 1942 with the much larger German warships *Lutzow* and *Admiral Hipper*. Apart from a few forays into the North Sea destroying German coastal convoys and patrolling on the Atlantic west of Ireland, Yogi's time on *Matabele* was uneventful but very happy. "I was sorry indeed to leave this ship," he wrote. "I liked everyone and would not have minded staying there." Fortunately, as it turned out, his next appointment was back to the "big ships," to the legendary battle cruiser HMS *Hood*, for the completion of his midshipman's education. *Matabele* was torpedoed and sunk off North Cape (Norway) on January 17, 1942. There were no survivors.

Hood was the largest (42,100 tons) and arguably the most handsome warship in the world. During the twenties particularly, *Hood* had proudly "shown the flag" in dozens of foreign ports, epitomizing British naval and imperial power. Shortly after Jenson joined the ship at Scapa Flow she was ordered to Rosyth, where some of her armour plate was removed to compensate for the installation of heavy new RDF (radar) and other electronic equipment, the addition of which would reduce *Hood*'s stability in heavy weather, a vital attribute of battle cruiser design.

Most of the time that spring, the midshipmen in *Hood* were exempted from other duties so that they could be further instructed in seamanship, gunnery, navigation, engineering, and other naval subjects, and so prepare for their acting sub-lieutenant's promotion examinations. Yogi passed these with distinction in April and was posted off *Hood* as a result. Those of his term-mates who failed the exams remained on board and were lost when the ship blew up and sank in an early morning gun battle on May 24, 1941, with the very powerful German battleship *Bismarck* and the heavy cruiser *Prinz Eugen* in the Denmark Strait west of Iceland. Only three of fifteen hundred British sailors survived. *Hood* and *Matabele* gone in a flash: Yogi Jenson had an undeniably charmed life.

He spent the rest of the spring and summer of 1941 on sub-lieutenants' courses in Portsmouth at the Royal Navy Torpedo School (HMS *Vernon*), the RN Gunnery School at Whale Island (HMS *Excellent*), and the RN Navigation School (HMS *Dryad*). In September 1941, his promotion to sub-lieutenant was confirmed. He was appointed to the Royal Canadian Navy after leave to Calgary, just over three years after he had left home.

After his leave, back in Halifax in late October 1941, Yogi was appointed to the River class destroyer HMCS *Ottawa*, which was based in St. John's, Newfoundland, as part of the newly formed Newfoundland Escort Force (NEF). After an uneventful overnight passage to Port-aux-Basques, Newfoundland, on the SS *Caribou* and the long train trip across Newfoundland to St. John's, he reported to the captain, Commander Hugh Pullen (Tom Pullen's older brother) and was assigned duty as the ship's gunnery officer, signals officer, and RDF (radar) officer. The older Pullen ran a "taut ship," as the saying goes, and the ratings (the "lower deck") called him "Von Pullen." He was strict but admired by both officers and the lower deck, and went on to become a respected rear-admiral.

Warships, particularly small ships at war more than in peacetime, have been thought of in two distinctly different ways. A warship has been and still is described in terms of its specifications as catalogued for more than a hundred years now in the much respected *Jane's Fighting Ships*: displacement, dimensions, complement, armament, propulsion machinery, etc.

On the other hand, especially after long experience together, a warship (large or small) was referred to by its ship's company as if it were human and a woman. "She" was lauded, scolded, cursed, loved, and truly missed.

After her commissioning trials, the legendary Lord Louis Mountbatten said that his beloved destroyer, HMS *Kelly*, was "a lovely ship; beautiful manners; does what she's told without a murmur." There was more than great spirit in "a happy and an efficient ship." It had a soul. When the *Kelly* was lost in action, Mountbatten, in a moving farewell address to what was left of his crew, said, "Now she lies in fifteen hundred fathoms and with more than half our shipmates. If they had to die, what a grand way to go, for now they all lie together in the ship we loved."[66] Soldiers and airmen had no similar emotional attachment to inanimate objects like tanks or bombers. Young people today can't conceive of such a feeling.

During the late nineteenth century, well before the development of the submarine as an effective weapon of war, the Whitehead self-propelled torpedo was launched from eighty- to one-hundred-ton "torpedo boats." A daring surprise attack in February 1904 by a flotilla of these tiny ships of the Japanese Navy sank or crippled several Russian battleships in the roadstead of Port Arthur in Manchuria. This and similar engagements seemed to require the development of heavier and faster "torpedo boat destroyers." With the First World War, they became just plain "destroyers" and were predominantly fleet escorts. They persisted in this role until the Second World War and the enormity of unrestricted submarine warfare necessitated the development of effective anti-submarine weapons and precise detection methods.

Between the wars, the basic design and function of the destroyer remained the same, but by the 1929–30 naval building programs, the displacement had inched up to twelve to fourteen hundred tons. The "V" and "W" class destroyers of First World War vintage and the destroyers built in the twenties and early thirties were equipped with four standard 4.7-inch guns and eight torpedo tubes in two quadruple mounts. This armament was completely appropriate for ships that would carry out lightning torpedo attacks against large enemy warships.

From its inception in 1910, the Royal Canadian Navy was a small dependent arm of the Royal Navy, and until 1929 all RCN ships were "retreads" from the Admiralty. Then Commodore Walter Hose succeeded in getting approval from his political masters in Ottawa for two brand new purpose-built destroyers, *Skeena* and *Saguenay*, both completed in the U.K. in 1931. These ships had two distinct advantages over conventional

RN destroyers: their hulls were specially strengthened against ice and they had steam heat for the Canadian winters.

The Naval Estimates of 1929 planned the construction of eight so-called "C" class destroyers of 1,375 tons displacement, but because of the financial drought of the Great Depression, the Admiralty had to pull in its horns and only four could be built: *Cygnet, Crescent, Comet,* and *Crusader.*

HMS *Crusader* (H 60) and her sister ship HMS *Comet* (H 00) were laid down in 1930 at Portsmouth Dockyard, and both were launched on September 30, 1931. Upon commissioning and working up, both *Crusader* and *Comet* joined the 2nd Destroyer Flotilla of the Royal Navy's Home Fleet. They spent the next six years in uneventful peacetime duty in British waters.

In 1936, the government of Canada negotiated with the Admiralty for the transfer of *Cygnet* (which became HMCS *St. Laurent*) and *Crescent* (which became HMCS *Fraser*) to replace two old Royal Navy castoffs, the destroyers *Champlain* and *Vancouver,* which were ready for the scrap heap. Our government wanted the Royal Navy to let us have *Crusader* and *Comet* on the same terms, but the Admiralty demurred. They would, however, sell these two ships to us.

After being taken in hand for the necessary refits at the Chatham Dockyard, both ships were commissioned into the Royal Canadian Navy on June 15, 1938. HMS *Comet* became HMCS *Restigouche* and HMS *Crusader* became HMCS *Ottawa.* On September 6, 1938, both sailed for their new home in Canada, Esquimalt, British Columbia, arriving there uneventfully on November 7.

In the last days of May 1939, the four ships escorted Their Majesties, King George VI and Queen Elizabeth, during their crossing from Vancouver to Victoria. Then on August 31, with Nazi Germany set to pounce on Poland, *St. Laurent* and *Fraser* were ordered to the east coast. Britain declared war on September 3 and Canada followed suit on September 10.

Early in the war, there were senior people at the Admiralty in London who seemed to regard the RCN as a sort of colonial clone of the Royal Navy and felt that our six little destroyers should become a squadron in some great imperial fleet. It took Prime Minister Mackenzie King's determined resistance to nip this notion in the bud and keep Canadian warships guarding Canada. RCN Permanent Force officers felt that ships like *Ottawa* armed with guns and torpedo tubes were designed for fleet surface engagements

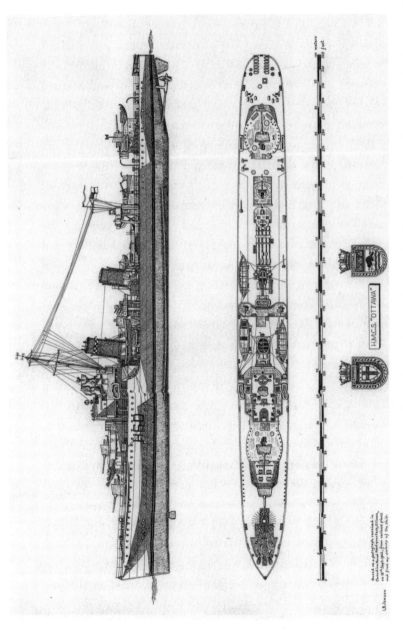

Line drawing of HMCS Ottawa by L.B. Jenson, "based on a photograph received at Canadian Naval Headquarters in Ottawa on 18 September 1942, from various plans and from my memory of the ship." (Courtesy of L.B. Jenson.)

and were never intended for hunting down and destroying submarines. However, we were faced with a critical shortage of convoy escort vessels and this was only partly relieved by our gaining seven of the fifty old American "flush deck" destroyers acquired through the famous "Ships for Bases" agreement brokered by Churchill and Roosevelt in December 1940.

Rear-Admiral Percy Nelles, the chief of naval staff, had nurtured the dream of building several of the new larger Tribal class destroyers in Canada. It became rapidly apparent that the construction of sophisticated warships like these was beyond the capacity of Canadian shipbuilding yards. However, the mass production of corvettes was not.

By early 1941, this national shipbuilding effort had been so successful that there were now more of these little ships being commissioned than there were men to man them. Most of their complement consisted of RCNVR officers and ratings with a few weeks of training at best. New corvettes were going to sea with the captain and a couple of petty officers the only members of the crew with any experience of shiphandling and none at all of anti-submarine weapons or warfare. Accordingly, the Royal Canadian Navy's performance in defending convoys from the U-boat scourge in the first three years of the war depended on necessarily rapid on-the-job training and was given a failing grade by senior Royal Navy officers.

In 1940, all British and Canadian destroyers were employed where they were most needed: fleet surface action duties in the ill-fated Norwegian campaign, assisting the evacuations from France, bombarding shore installations, and so on. The most recently built class, the Tribals, had been designed for Jutland-type fleet engagements in the North Sea. They had a short range that had to be significantly increased for operations in the North Atlantic later on. As the danger from submarines and aircraft became more intense, the older destroyers lost half their torpedo tubes and a three-inch high angle anti-aircraft gun replaced one of the surface weapons. More depth charge throwers were fitted and more depth charges stowed on the upper deck.

At least in the beginning, this was a one-ocean war, and so, on November 15, 1939, *Ottawa* and *Restigouche* were ordered to the east coast, reaching Halifax on December 7, 1939. TC-1,[67] the first troop convoy to leave Canada, was escorted out of the Halifax approaches by *Fraser*, *Restigouche*, *St. Laurent*, and *Ottawa* on December 10. The 7,400 men of

First Canadian Division were carried on board the liners *Aquitania, Empress of Britain, Duchess of Bedford, Monarch of Bermuda,* and *Empress of Australia.*

In April 1940, *Ottawa* suffered extensive damage to her stem when she collided with the tug *Bansurf* and was *hors de combat* until June 12. Accordingly, when the British government asked on May 23, 1940, for all available RCN destroyers to assist in the defence against possible German invasion, *Ottawa* was unable to join *Skeena, Restigouche, Fraser,* and *St. Laurent.*

She finally got her orders to proceed overseas escorting another troop convoy, TC-7, arriving at Greenock, Scotland, on September 4, 1940, after an uneventful crossing. Much of her early duty involved acting as escort during the initial stage of a convoy's passage out of harbour. However, there were rather more eventful moments.

At 1945 hours of November 4, 1940, after escorting yet another convoy, WS-4, out of Liverpool, *Ottawa,* with Commander (later Vice-Admiral) Rollo Mainguy her fourth commanding officer, was ordered along with the destroyer HMS *Harvester* to go to the aid of the merchant ship *Melrose Abbey* some 150 miles distant, which had reported that she was being shelled by a submarine on the surface. The two destroyers dashed in at thirty-four knots and fired five salvoes at the crash-diving sub, unfortunately without making any hits. Then, in nine separate attacks, they fired and dropped seventy-three depth charges. A very large oil slick was seen and the Admiralty credited the two hunters with "probably damaging" an as-yet-unidentified submarine but not with a kill. Some time later, the sleuths at Admiralty Intelligence determined that a relatively new Italian submarine, *Commandante Faa' Di Bruno,* had been lost in roughly the same location on November 6, 1940. Much later, in 1982, it was confirmed that this submarine had indeed been sunk by *Ottawa* and *Harvester,* making it the first RCN sub kill of the war.

From November 1940 to June 1941, *Ottawa* took on repeated routine convoy escort duties. Then, on June 5, along with other Canadian destroyers operating in United Kingdom waters, she was ordered to join the newly formed Newfoundland Escort Force based at St. John's.

The first real test of the new force came on June 20, 1941, with Convoy HX-133, consisting of forty-eight ships escorted by *Ottawa,* the corvettes

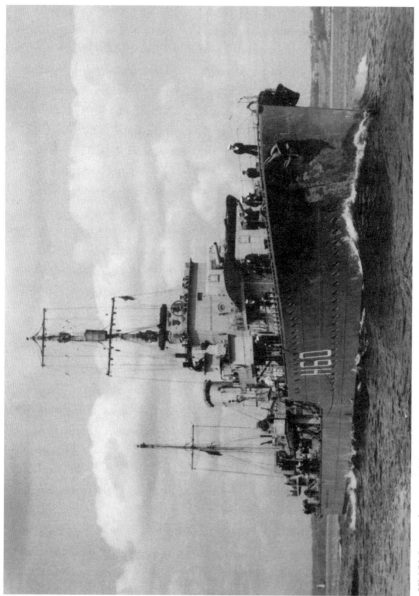

HMCS Ottawa leaving Halifax Harbour, September 1940. (Courtesy of Public Archives of Canada H206.)

Chambly, Collingwood, and *Orillia,* and the armed merchant cruiser HMS *Wolfe.* Ten U-boats converged on it, led by U-203, and quickly sank eight ships without any significant response on the part of the escort vessels.

But then finally at 0024 hours of June 27, *Ottawa* got a clear contact and dropped a full pattern of depth charges. Then she lost contact despite a thorough search. Newly joined corvette HMS *Nasturtium* regained the contact at 0735, which she was able to hold until, at 1258, a mortally wounded U-boat broke surface and sank after being abandoned by its crew. This proved to be U-556, commanded by Kapitän-Leutnant Wohlfarth, reputed to be one of the ranking German submarine aces.

On June 8, 1941, just before *Ottawa* led the escort group for convoy HX-133 out of St. John's, Warrant Officer Lloyd Irwin Jones joined her as its gunner (T) (torpedo gunner). From his memoirs, it's clear that young Yogi Jenson thought a lot of this man: "Our Gunner (T) was Mr. Lloyd Jones, promoted from the ranks and given a Warrant, a type of commission with the full status of a commissioned officer. Many of these gentlemen were later promoted to Lieutenant and higher; some even made Admiral! I have to say that I really admired Lloyd Jones, an 'old man' of 32 versus my 21 years. What a fine, wise, experienced gentleman he was!"[68]

Jones had joined the peacetime RCN as a boy seaman in May 1929 and had worked his way up through the lower deck ranks to chief petty officer in June 1940. He was given his warrant (a form of commission from the ranks) as acting gunner (T) in April 1941 and was posted to HMS *Vernon,* the Royal Navy Torpedo School at Portsmouth, for advanced training in depth charge technology, a critical skill at that time in the Battle of the Atlantic. Then, on June 8, 1941, Lloyd Jones was posted to *Ottawa.*

After a major refit requiring repairs to storm-damaged screws (propellers) in Saint John, New Brunswick, was completed on September 16, 1941, *Ottawa* rejoined NEF at St. John's and resumed her escort duties. Over the next four months, several convoys were escorted without incident.

In early November, just after young Sub-Lieutenant Jenson had joined the ship, *Ottawa* proceeded to Halifax for repairs to her ASDIC dome. While she was there, a fresh draft of ratings was taken on. One of them, Sid Dobing, had seen almost as much action as Yogi Jenson. Young Sid hailed from Edson, Alberta, and, together with a like-minded friend (who was

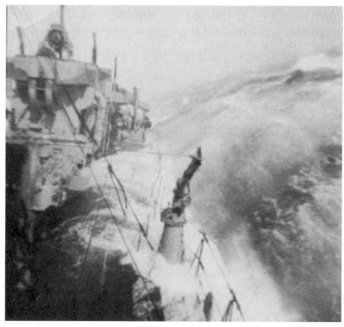

Ottawa *in heavy mid-Atlantic seas, 1941. (Courtesy of George Beveridge.)*

killed early in the war), decided to head overseas to the U.K. before the declaration of war in September 1939 and enlist in the Royal Navy, as joining
the RCN was just going to take too long. He trained as a boy seaman and
was drafted three months later (still a boy seaman) to one of the new Tribal
class destroyers, HMS *Mashona*. His first taste of action was during the
abortive Allied Expeditionary Force landing and evacuation in the
Norwegian campaign in April–June 1940, when his ship was repeatedly
bombed but escaped unscathed.

> The next major action occurred in May 1941 when in
> company with HMS *Rodney*, a British battleship, we
> became involved in the hunt for the German battleship
> *Bismarck*, which had sunk the battlecruiser HMS *Hood*.
> We stayed with the *Rodney* during the chase and subse-
> quent engagement. During the battle, I had the good for-
> tune to spend one hour on the bridge as a lookout and had
> a ringside seat during the battle. That was the only time in
> my naval career that I was overwhelmed by offers to take

my place. The *Bismarck* was eventually on fire from stem to stern and finally sank with a very heavy loss of life. At the time we considered it revenge for the loss of so many lives on the *Hood,* when she was sunk just a few days before. Later on we realized that the enemy sailors were just like us, doing a job that they had been given. Another one of the great tragedies of war.

Mashona and her sister ship the *Tartar* were ordered to head for Plymouth upon completion of the action, as both ships were very low on fuel.… The next day the German Air Force located the two destroyers (off the southern coast of Ireland) and commenced a bombing attack that … resulted in hits on the *Mashona.* There was heavy damage and it was soon evident that the ship could not be saved.… *Tartar* picked up all of the survivors, and … we were taken to Greenock on the Clyde and from there to the barracks in Chatham. Shortly after returning from survivors leave I was informed that I would be transferred to the Royal Canadian Navy, if I was willing to do so. My parents had learned that they could request a transfer, as I was still under 21 and apparently they were entitled to make the request. Although I was happy in the Royal Navy I jumped at the chance of returning to Canada and soon found myself on a troop ship, bound for Halifax. On arrival, I was granted leave and returned to my hometown, Edson, Alberta, where my parents were still residing and where I had attended school. On completion of my leave I returned to *Stadacona,* where I completed a Seaman Torpedoman course, following which I was drafted to HMCS *Ottawa.*[69]

Michael Barriault was another draftee who'd had a brush with danger at sea before joining *Ottawa.* He'd been raised in Curling, Newfoundland, and in 1938, at age seventeen, went to sea on the SS *Humber Arm,* a newsprint and passenger ship owned by the Bowaters Pulp and Paper Company with some boys from the Bay of Islands region, including a friend named Frank Morrison. During the next two years on board, he trained as a ship's steward. On July 13, 1940, the ship was torpedoed and sunk off the Irish coast. After this, Michael returned to Canada, enlisted in the Royal Canadian Navy, and after some months working at Admiralty House in HMC Dockyard, Halifax, he was drafted to HMCS *Ottawa* as a leading steward. There he discovered his friend Frank Morrison, who had been in *Ottawa* since June 1941 as a stoker.

Alvin Underhill was on board as well. At age nineteen, he was just out of school in rural New Brunswick, and upon entry into the navy he had been sent for basic training clear across Canada to HMCS *Naden* in Victoria, British Columbia. He was one of twenty-five ordinary seamen drafted to HMCS *Ottawa* in August 1941 when the ship was in Saint John, New Brunswick, for repairs and refit. Only five of the original group of twenty-five survived the sinking of *Ottawa* on September 13, 1942.

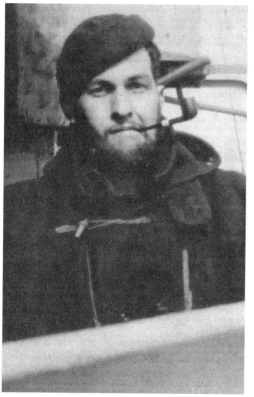

Able Seaman C.R. "Roe" Skillen on the bridge of HMCS Ottawa, *May 1942. (Courtesy of Susan Skillen Joseph.)*

George Johnson was a plumbing apprentice and naval reservist in Burlington, Ontario, when he was called up for active service in May 1941. After five months of indoctrination at HMCS *Star* in Hamilton, he was sent on to HMCS *Stadacona* in late October 1941 to learn the rudiments of being a stoker. A little over two months later, on January 6, 1942, he was drafted to *Ottawa*. Just like so many other ratings, George Johnson has fond memories of several brief but friendly conversations he had with "Surgeon Lieutenant Hendry" on the upper deck.

Roe Skillen came down from Keewatin in Northern Ontario, and after working on a survey crew for a period of time on the CPR (someone told him that would assure him of a railway job after the war) he enlisted in the navy in June 1940. He had some commissioning time in the corvette HMCS *Saskatoon*, and following QR3 rating gunnery courses at HMCS *Stadacona*, he joined *Ottawa* at Halifax in June 1941.

When *Ottawa*'s repairs were completed on November 19, she sailed for St. John's and joined a thirty-six-ship convoy, SC 57, on November 29 on its eastbound run. On the night of December 1, strong headwinds and snowstorms forced the convoy to heave to, and two of its ships, *Csiskos* and *Empire Cabot*, subjected to heavy weather damage, had to return to St. John's. The remainder of the convoy limped on, and *Ottawa* detached near Iceland. On December 10, the convoy was attacked 325 miles west-north-west of Donegal and three ships, *Kurdistan*, *Kirnwood*, and *Star of Luxor*, were torpedoed and sunk within minutes. After a five-day layover in Iceland, *Ottawa* joined the westbound convoy ON 46, of twenty-eight ships, on December 16 and returned to Newfoundland.

On December 21, 1941, Commander Pullen was relieved as captain by Commander C.D. ("Do") Donald, a man of impressive athletic build who had been one of the navy's champion sportsmen. Then, *Ottawa* took over as SOE (Senior Officer of the Escort) for the thirty-ship convoy SC 64, which she joined on January 10, 1942. That night, a fierce gale struck, and the destroyer lost visual contact with the other escorting corvettes and indeed the entire convoy. The oscillator for *Ottawa*'s ASDIC was so badly damaged that she was obliged to return to St. John's for its urgent replacement. On January 13, with *Ottawa* absent, the convoy was attacked, and the 5,441-ton *Friar Rock* was torpedoed and sunk with only seven survivors. The repair job done, *Ottawa* rejoined the convoy that same day, but the rest of the eastward run was marked by continuing rough weather and poor visibility.

In February, during refuelling off Moville (Loch Foyle), Sub-Lieutenant L.B. Jenson was involved in an incident that he recorded faithfully many years later.[70] The captain's day cabin flat was accidentally flooded with oil, which precipitated the captain, Commander Do Donald, out of his bath, "large, hairy and pink," and which sent young Jenson scurrying up to the upper deck to evade the mess. The ship was ordered to Belfast for repairs and for the installation of much-needed additional depth charge throwers. While this was being accomplished, Yogi was flown over to Campbeltown in Scotland for an overdue anti-submarine warfare course.

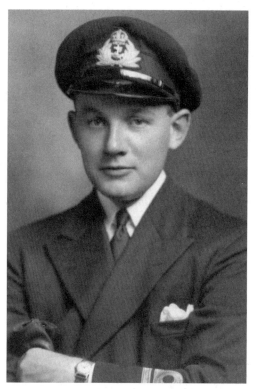

Lieutenant T.C. "Tom" Pullen, Ottawa's *twenty-four-year-old first lieutenant (executive officer), one of sixty-nine rescued members of the ship's company. (Courtesy of Elizabeth Pullen.)*

On February 17, 1942, Lieutenant Thomas Charles Pullen, RCN, was appointed *Ottawa's* first lieutenant (executive officer), joining the ship in Belfast while she was undergoing the refit and repairs. Tom Pullen was born on May 27, 1918, into a military family in Oakville, Ontario, the youngest of three sons and two daughters. His eldest brother, Hugh, had just been captain of *Ottawa* and went on to reach flag rank as a rear-admiral. His middle brother, Duff, served overseas as an officer in the Lorne Scots and rose to be its colonel. Tom attended Lakefield School from 1929 to 1935. By that time, he was determined to go into the navy. Tom spent one year at Oakville High School, where the principal, Mr. Archibald, prepared him for the Royal Navy officer cadet entrance examination. At that time, Lakefield "put much emphasis on sports and outdoor activities and Tom said he'd never have passed the exams in that setting."[71] He sailed in RMS *Ansonia* to the U.K. with seven other candidates in August 1936. His training began on September 9, 1936, at Portsmouth in HMS *Frobisher* and was identical to Yogi Jenson's. In May 1937, he trained in two RN cruisers, *Shropshire* and *Sussex,* and two destroyers, *Hotspur* and *Hostile.* On October 23, 1939, Tom Pullen was promoted sub-lieutenant and appointed to his first Canadian ship, HMCS *Assiniboine.* In January 1985, he could look back on that time with considerable affection:

> I can remember … going down to Plymouth from HMS *Excellent* [the Royal Navy Gunnery School] on the outbreak of war in 1939 to join my first Canadian ship. I'd

been in the Navy 3 years by then … HMCS *Assiniboine* [was] commissioning there, and Commander [later Vice-Admiral] E.R. Mainguy was the captain…. He is one man for whom I have a great deal of respect … even now, the memory of my time in that ship … he taught us a great deal." Hennessy [later VAdm RL Hennessy, DSC, RCN] and Pullen were the sub-lieutenants "and it was great fun, it was a great learning process…. You had to learn fast in those days because the Navy was expanding and there were not enough experienced and trained officers to go around … so prospects were bright and it paid to pay attention![72]

On May 15, 1940, T.C. Pullen was promoted lieutenant and, in January 1941, took a specialty course at the Whale Island Gunnery School (HMS *Excellent*) in Portsmouth. In November 1941, he was appointed executive officer, and then, on February 1, 1942, commanding officer of HMCS *Niobe*, the Canadian shore establishment in Scotland. Finally, Pullen was appointed first lieutenant to *Ottawa*, which he joined in Belfast on February 17. At that point, Tom was just twenty-four years old.

The repair work completed, *Ottawa* proceeded to Greenock in Scotland and finally sailed from the Clyde on February 23, 1942. Yogi Jenson remembers that trip back all too well:

We were heading back to St. John's when the weather changed dramatically. We ran into a heavy westerly gale and soon were heading into towering seas, with huge waves 60 feet or more in height. The troughs were deep and seemed sheltered from the wind. The ship would then climb the next monster wave. Finally at the top, the sea looked like the dawn of creation, an awesome view of great mounds of water, all striped with greybeards, long lines of foam. Then down into the trough again, and so it went, on and on. From time to time, waves would sweep down the upper deck forcing anyone there to grab the lifeline and hold on for dear life. For almost five days, the ship steamed ahead at 12 knots, but actually went astern about 200 miles over the ground![73]

The accumulated weather damage to the ship was so bad that when she put in to Halifax on March 15, she was deemed unfit to carry out even coastal escort duties. The RDF (radar) was out of order, the forward 4.7-inch shell magazine had been flooded, and the stanchions between the lower and the upper messdecks had been badly banged about. The necessary major repairs took until May 22, 1942, to complete.

George Hendry was appointed to HMCS *Stadacona*, the shore base in Halifax, on February 20, 1942, and joined *Ottawa* when it returned there on March 17. Yogi Jenson recalls:

> As always was the case at that time [when a ship was in port for refit or repairs] there was a substantial reappointment of officers and drafting of men to other ships or shore duties. Our surgeon was among those appointed elsewhere and he was relieved by Surgeon Lieutenant George Hendry ... a quiet, very sober and scholarly gentleman compared with his predecessor. I was impressed favourably with Dr. Hendry and found him to be an agreeable messmate with whom I could enjoy conversation. Of course, I had no idea of how he carried out his medical duties but I believe the other officers and the ship's company wholeheartedly shared my opinion that he was very capable.
>
> I was particularly impressed with Dr. Hendry when a young seaman in my RDF section had an epileptic fit in the messdeck while I was passing by. Evidently, these fits had occurred before but his messmates piled on to him and held him down until the fit subsided. In this case, I sent one of the men aft to bring the doctor. Lieutenant Hendry arrived very quickly and knelt beside the man who was still convulsing. Hendry whispered in the man's ear and immediately the convulsions ceased. The man got to his feet, none the worse for wear. Later in the ward room, I asked the doctor what he had done to restore the man and he said "I hypnotized him." When I asked where he had learned to do that, he told me that it was in medical school. I certainly didn't think he was joking. He seemed very serious.[74]

Though they became good friends, George never said a word about his wife, and Yogi knew nothing of Betty Summers. This was not surprising to Jenson at the time or since, as particularly during the war, naval officers kept their personal lives to themselves. On one occasion, however, George did confide to Yogi about his vulnerability to alcohol:

> One evening, I think it was after a mess dinner, when most of us in the ward room had had more than enough to drink, I noticed that George Hendry was very sober. When I asked him why he seemed not to drink like the rest of us, he replied that alcohol had a bad effect on him. Some evening later, one of our officers persuaded him to have a few glasses. He did and it certainly seemed to make him completely different. He laughingly told me that this was what liquor did to him. I never saw him take a drink of spirits again.[75]

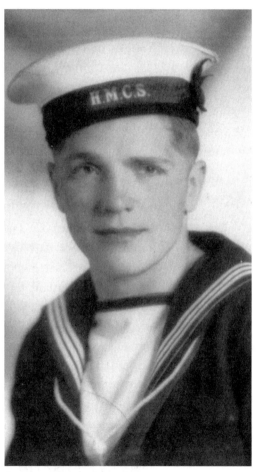

AB George Beveridge had joined *Ottawa* in the summer of 1941 after serving in the ex-USN four-stacker *St. Clair* but missed *Ottawa*'s sinking by a bit of luck. When *Ottawa* required a major refit in Halifax between April 29 and May 22, 1942, he was sent temporarily to Port Arthur, Ontario (now Thunder Bay), as crew for a newly commissioned Bangor class minesweeper, *Fort William*. This ship was in the Gulf of St. Lawrence

Boy Seaman Steve Logos, age seventeen. He joined the navy on June 2, 1941: "Pay was 50 cents a day. No tot of rum as too young." (Courtesy of Steve Logos.)

en route to Halifax when *Ottawa* was sunk. George Beveridge thought George Hendry "a great human being.... As an officer he was always available for a casual or a serious talk.... In short, he was a doctor first and a naval officer second."[76]

Edward Fox joined the navy straight out of high school in December 1941. He was posted to *Stadacona* for training as an ASDIC operator and was drafted to *Ottawa* at some point in late spring 1942.

Steve Logos had been raised by his father from early childhood in Calgary, Alberta, as his parents had separated soon after he was born.

> I had just finished high school, had written my finals early and was in Victoria, B.C., for new entry training on June 2nd, 1941. A little fuzzy-cheeked kid going off to war and maybe becoming a hero.... After new entry training was finished, I went home for two weeks' leave and then it was five nights and four days on the train to Halifax.
>
> Within a couple of days, I was drafted to an old four-funneled ex-USN lend-lease destroyer, HMCS *Hamilton*, and it took me all of three months to get over my sea-sickness. Even at that, every time I went to sea again, I would feel woozy the first day. They took me off that one and put me on HMCS *Columbia* (another of the same type) for three months. Then, because they needed qualified tradesmen, I was sent ashore for a torpedoman's course. Besides torpedoes, we had to look after depth charges and some of the electrical equipment, and we had to stand watch.
>
> I joined the *Ottawa* at the end of May 1942. She was one of the better destroyers in the Royal Canadian Navy. We lived in very tight quarters. There were 18 of us in the torpedomen's mess, which was all of 300 square feet. We slept in hammocks in the mess, we ate in the mess, we wrote letters, played cards and stowed all our gear in lockers in the mess. And it was imperative that it be kept clean. Under these conditions, you had to get along with everybody in the mess regardless and many great friendships did develop amongst the fellows.

We had a full fledged doctor aboard our ship, Surgeon Lieutenant George Hendry. He was a very gentle man and a real favourite with those of us in the lower deck. He would come around and spend quite a bit of time talking to us.[77]

For hundreds of years, there had existed a yawning social gap in the Royal Navy between officers and men of the lower deck, and this sort of stratification was inevitably passed on to the RCN through Canadian naval officers who had trained in the RN before the war. George Hendry did a lot to break down this barrier by his warm and caring relationship with the ratings in *Ottawa*, and they never forgot it.

Ordinary Seaman Joseph Terrabassi, V19351, had had a rough start in life and almost seemed like an orphan out of a Dickens novel. Not surprisingly, he was (and still is) known to all as "Terry." Born June 3, 1923, in Timmins, Ontario, he was eleven when his parents separated, and he lived with his mother until she died from tuberculosis one year later. His father would not take him in but paid for twelve-year-old Terry to live in various boarding houses. Then, after a further year, his father died, and he went to live with relatives in Belle River, Ontario, near Windsor. A further two years on, he quit Grade 8 and began to work as a butcher's apprentice to earn enough to support himself.

When the war came Terry wanted to join the navy at age seventeen. His aunt refused to sign the consent papers, so Terry had to wait until his eighteenth birthday, June 3, 1941. After basic training

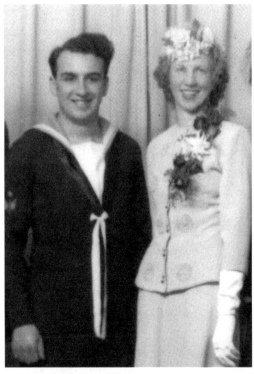

Terry and Millie Terrabassi on their wedding day, April 19, 1943. (Courtesy of Terry Terrabassi.)

in Windsor, he was posted to HMCS *Stadacona* in Halifax, where he completed his Radar I course in early March 1942. He was drafted to HMCS *Ottawa* in April and was promoted able seaman in August just before the ship's last eastbound convoy run. At age nineteen, he was on his own, and though he had virtually no ties with the shore, he was healthy and he had a trade, even if operating a radar set was a bit of a stretch from cutting meat.

Terry Terrabassi agreed with Steve Logos, Alvin Underhill, Sid Dobing, and the other ratings of *Ottawa's* lower deck: George Hendry was a kind, decent man and a very good doctor. Certainly, he was not the typical aloof RCN officer. You could talk to him and he would listen.

Able Seaman Norm Wilson was born in Vancouver, B.C., on March 8, 1921. "I enlisted in the navy on September 20, 1939, and went on active service in August 1940." After taking preliminary gunnery training, he was posted to an armed yacht, HMCS *Cougar*, doing coastal patrol, as Norm says, " in and out of every inlet and cove on Vancouver Island." In March 1942, he was posted to HMCS *Stadacona* in Halifax for advanced training as a QR II gunnery rating and then joined *Ottawa* in St. John's, Newfoundland, on May 23, 1942. They made a couple of uneventful convoy runs before Ottawa's last run westward in September.[78] Even though Norm was in *Ottawa* for barely four months before she was lost, he agreed with his messmates that George Hendry was certainly not "your usual standoffish RCN officer."

Lieutenant Dunn Lantier, who joined *Ottawa* in late May 1942, had not taken his training as a naval officer cadet overseas with the Royal Navy as Yogi Jenson, Tom Pullen, and Larry Rutherford had. Lantier grew up in Montreal, the son of a prominent dental surgeon, had been sent to two prestigious private schools, and had then gone on to the Royal Military College in Kingston, where he graduated in 1938. Lantier had all of his naval officer cadet training during the summers of 1934–38 at HMCS *Stadacona* in Halifax and on board the destroyer HMCS *Saguenay*, When he gained his promotion to lieutenant in 1939, he was appointed to be the aide-de-camp to two governors-general of Canada, first to Lord Tweedsmuir (who as John Buchan was the author of *The Thirty-Nine Steps*) and, following Tweedsmuir's death in 1940, to the Earl of Athlone. In 1941–42, Lantier had been trained in anti-submarine warfare (HMC

A/S School) and then served briefly in the Royal Navy destroyer HMS *Vanquisher* before joining *Ottawa* in May.

On May 29, 1942, the repairs completed, *Ottawa* joined the sixty-two-ship convoy SC 85 as SOE (Senior Officer of the Escort). This was certainly a slow convoy, with an average speed of 6.9 knots, but the weather was good, the enemy was not encountered, and all ships arrived safely. The return westward run with ON 105 (thirty-six ships) was made from June 19 to 30 without incident.

In late June, the ship's company was assembled on *Ottawa's* foredeck for what proved to be their last group photograph. Too many of the men in this photograph were lost when the ship was sunk on September 13, 1942.

Commander Do Donald was relieved by Acting Lieutenant-Commander Clark Anderson Rutherford, RCN, on July 5, 1942, and went on to command the new naval repair base at Shelburne, Nova Scotia. Larry Rutherford was twenty-eight years old at the time, and his performance to date had been impressive, so much so that it was put about that he was certainly headed to flag rank. After a year at Royal Military College in Kingston, Ontario, he took passage to Britain on September 1, 1933, to begin his training as a naval officer cadet on board HMS *Frobisher* in Portsmouth, similar to that of Yogi Jenson and Tom Pullen.

After a year, he was promoted midshipman and served in three old battleships (*Resolution, Revenge,* and *Royal Sovereign*), a cruiser (*Berwick*), and a destroyer (*Brazen*) with the Mediterranean Fleet and on the China Station. Throughout most of 1937, he finished the requisite courses at the Royal Naval College, Greenwich, in HMS *Excellent* (Whale Island) gunnery school and in HMS *Dryad,* the navigation school. On December 19, 1937, he was appointed as a sub-lieutenant to the recently commissioned destroyer HMCS *Fraser* (ex-HMS *Crescent*), then stationed on the west coast of Canada. Rutherford was promoted lieutenant on May 15, 1938. With war looming on August 31, 1939, *Fraser* and *St. Laurent* were ordered to the Atlantic coast "with all dispatch." Canada declared war on September 10, 1939 (one week after Great Britain), as *Fraser* was transiting the Panama Canal. She was based in Halifax until spring, escorting some of the earliest convoys and patrolling against possible enemy surface raiders.

On April 1, 1940, Rutherford was appointed first lieutenant to the River class destroyer HMCS *Skeena,* which was also based in Halifax.

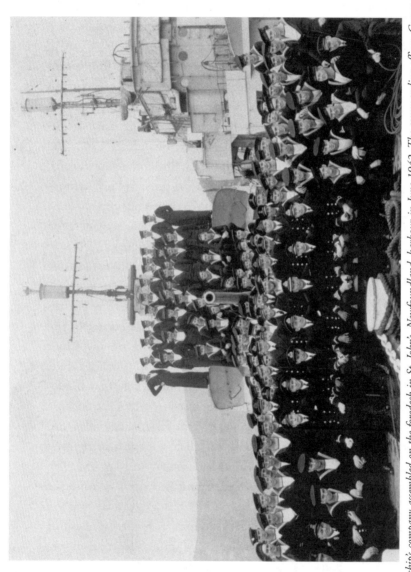

Ottawa's ship's company assembled on the foredeck in St. John's, Newfoundland, harbour in June 1942. The commanding officer, Commander C.D. Donald, is seated centre front row, with Lieutenant T.C. Pullen to his right. Commander Donald was relieved as captain by Lieutenant-Commander C.A. "Larry" Rutherford on July 5, 1942. (Courtesy of Public Archives of Canada FN 532 and Marilyn Gurney, Curator of Maritime Command Museum, Admiralty House, HMCS Stadacona, Halifax.)

With the German invasion of France, four RCN destroyers (*Skeena, St. Laurent, Restigouche,* and *Fraser*) were ordered overseas, again "with all dispatch," for convoy escort duties. With U-boats operating increasingly westward in 1941, the Newfoundland Escort Force (NEF) was formed out of St. John's. *Skeena* joined this force in June 1941 and began escorting convoys, initially as far as Iceland. On August 26, 1941, Lieutenant Rutherford was appointed to command the ex-USN four-stacker destroyer *St. Francis.* Again the duty was escorting transatlantic convoys, at first as far as Iceland, but then in early 1942 the NEF was reorganized

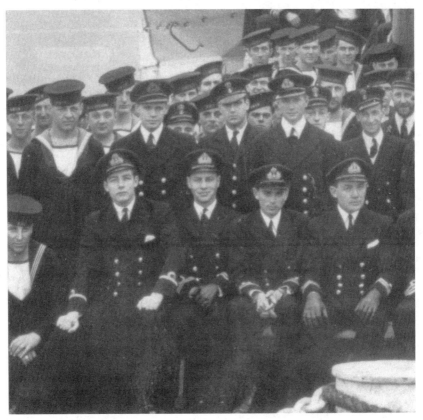

At the left end of the second row of this enlargement of the ship's company photograph (see opposite) is AB William "Pooch" Bucheski, who will be the appendectomy patient on September 7, 1942, and next to him is his surgeon, Surgeon Lieutenant George Hendry. On the far right of the second row is Leading Sick Berth Attendant Alexander MacMillan. At the left end of the front row is Sub-Lieutenant L.B. "Yogi" Jenson. Next to him is Lieutenant Dunn Lantier, and at the far right is First Lieutenant T.C. "Tom" Pullen.

as Mid-Ocean Escort Force (MOEF), shuttling between St. John's and Londonderry in Northern Ireland.

On June 15, 1942, Larry Rutherford was promoted to the acting rank of lieutenant commander at the age of twenty-eight. Following his appointment to command *Ottawa* on July 5, he took her through three completely uneventful convoy runs: HX 197 (twenty-four ships) on July 8, ON 116 (thirty-six ships) on July 25, and SC 96 (twenty-seven ships),

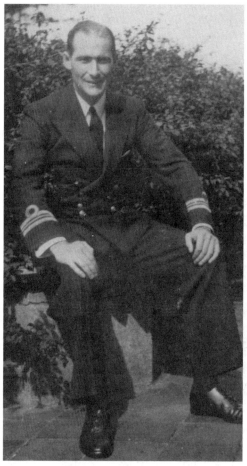

which was delivered intact on August 27, 1942. Thus, from November 19, 1941, to August 27, 1942, *Ottawa* had escorted 276 ships and only four of them were lost. In fact, three of these were sunk on the eastern leg of convoy SC 57's run, which *Ottawa* was not involved in.

The ship's company of *Ottawa* — the men who manned her, handled her, navigated her, "fought" her (as sailors in Nelson's day would have said) — were very young indeed. With the exception of the senior petty officers, most of the ratings were between the ages of eighteen and twenty-two, barely out of their teens.

Lieutenant Commander C.A. "Larry" Rutherford, Ottawa's twenty-eight-year-old captain who gave his lifebelt to a sailor who had none and was lost, exhausted after four days' continuous duty conning the ship. (Courtesy of Robert A. Rutherford.)

Captain Larry Rutherford was twenty-eight, First Lieutenant Tom Pullen was twenty-four, Sub-Lieutenant Yogi Jenson was twenty-one, and Surgeon Lieutenant George Hendry was thirty-one. At the ripe old age of thirty-two, one of the oldest men on the ship was Warrant Officer Lloyd Irwin Jones, the gunner (T)!

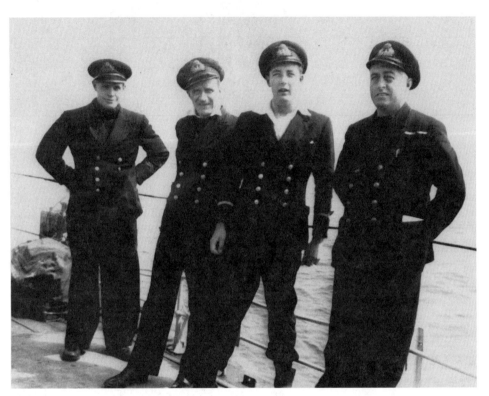

On the deck of Ottawa *during its last eastbound convoy run. Left to right: Surgeon Lieutenant G.A. Hendry, RCNVR; Lieutenant (E) John Somers, RCNR; Sub-Lieutenant L.B. Jenson, RCN; and Lieutenant P.M. Crawford, RCNR. Somers and Crawford were passengers in* Ottawa, *en route to take up commands in the U.K. This is the last photograph of George Hendry. (Courtesy of Elizabeth Pullen.)*

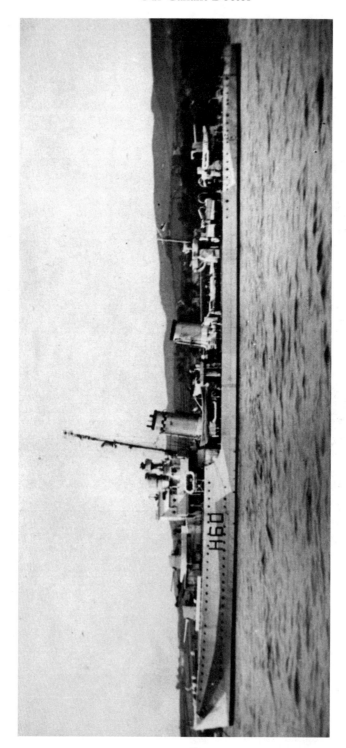

The last photograph of HMCS Ottawa lying in Lough Foyle, Northern Ireland, taken by Lieutenant T.C. Pullen on September 4, 1942, from a "skimmer" (a fourteen-foot planing boat used for despatches). The ship sailed the next day on its last (and fatal) convoy run. (Courtesy of Public Archives of Canada NF979.)

Into the Black Pit 5

5

At 0730 on September 5, 1942, Escort Group C-4 got underway for the forty-mile run down Lough Foyle to its rendezvous with Convoy ON 127 off Rathlin Island in the North Channel leading from the Irish Sea to the North Atlantic. C-4 was led by the old ex-USN four-stacker destroyer *St. Croix*,[79] with her captain, Lieutenant Commander Andrew H. "Dobby" Dobson, RCNR, as SOE. Also on the convoy were *Ottawa* (Lieutenant Commander C.A. Rutherford, RCN); three RCN corvettes, *Amherst* (Lieutenant H.G. Denyer, RCNR), *Arvida* (Lieutenant A.I. MacKay, RCNR), and *Sherbrooke* (Lieutenant J.A.M. Levesque, RCNR); and an RN corvette, *Celandine* (Lieutenant P.V. Collings, RNR). (See Appendix G.)

Ottawa had just completed a very brief layover and refit in Londonderry. During this time, the ratings (or the "troops," as Tom Pullen called them in his memoirs) had applied "a novel Western Approaches camouflage scheme of white and pale shades of blue and green" paint to the ship.[80] *Ottawa's* ratings always liked a layover in Londonderry. It was a friendly port town with nice girls and good beer, offering the men a chance to relax a bit. The hills down Lough Foyle were lush green and far from the war.

In late August, Surgeon Lieutenant George Hendry had obtained a short leave to take a rush trip by air (RAF "sked run") to London, where he had dinner with an old friend and medical classmate, Henry Swan. Then on to Bramshott (next to the famous Aldershot) to visit his old *Varsity* chum, classmate and hockey teammate Frank Shipp, a major in the Royal Canadian Army Medical Corps with the 15th Canadian General Hospital.[81] The hospital had been swamped on August 20 by the arrival of 230 wounded survivors of the Dieppe Raid (the day before) who had been landed from destroyers at Gosport (across Portsmouth harbour), transferred to the Royal Naval Hospital at nearby Haslar, and then moved quickly on to Bramshott. Many of these men were badly injured. Frank Shipp and his surgical and nursing colleagues had been operating day and night right up to George Hendry's visit on August 28.[82]

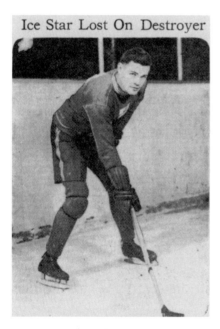

Ice Star Lost On Destroyer

"Ice star lost on destroyer," Toronto Evening Telegram, *Tuesday, September 22, 1942. The caption of the photograph reads: "Surgeon-Lieut. George Hendry, who captained the University of Toronto hockey team in 1934, is reported missing and believed killed. He was surgeon on the destroyer* Ottawa, *and had just recently visited a Varsity chum, Major Frank L. Shipp, in England."*

On September 4, the ship dropped down river to anchor off Moville (Eire). "After anchoring," Tom Pullen "went away in the 'skimmer' [a fourteen-foot planing boat used for dispatches] with the Sub [Sub-Lieutenant L.B. Jenson, RCN] and the Buffer [chief boatswain's mate], Petty Officer Smith, to admire the ship's company's handiwork from afar. With a borrowed camera, we took photographs, the last ever taken of our ship and treasured for that reason."[83] (See page 108.) And so they slipped down the forty miles of Lough Foyle to meet their convoy in the North Channel opposite Rathlin Island.

Lieutenant Commander Dobson's ship, *St. Croix*, was one of

fifty old retread so-called four-stacker destroyers of the United States Navy (and one of seven turned over to Canada) that were traded to Britain in exchange for bases in Newfoundland, Bermuda, and the British West Indies as part of a deal brokered by Churchill and Roosevelt in 1940. The United States Navy built 273 of these narrow beam ships in 1919–20 and then, for reasons of postwar economy, most of them were promptly consigned to the Reserve "mothball" Fleet until 1939. Along with five of her sister four-stackers, *St. Croix* was commissioned into the Royal Canadian Navy on September 24, 1940. These ships had been originally designed for service in the balmy Pacific, not in the blustery Atlantic. They were immediately taken for a refit to have heating units installed in order to make them even marginally bearable. They were also fitted with new depth charge and ASDIC apparatus that made them more top-heavy than they already were. Because of their narrow beam, these ships were notoriously difficult to handle even in light seas, and once, when crowned with tons of ice, *St. Croix* did come perilously close to capsizing.

She joined the Newfoundland Escort Force in August 1941, and in July 1942, as a member of Escort Group C-2 covering Convoy ON 113, she sank the German submarine U-90. This was a remarkable accomplishment, as C-2's six escort ships had either the poorest radar (Type 286M) or none at all. The ship's captain, Lieutenant Commander

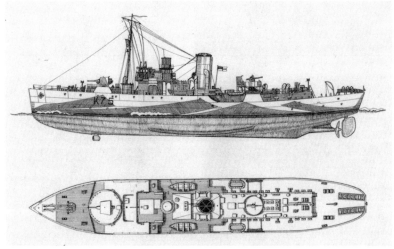

Line drawing of HMS Celandine, *by L.B. Jenson.*

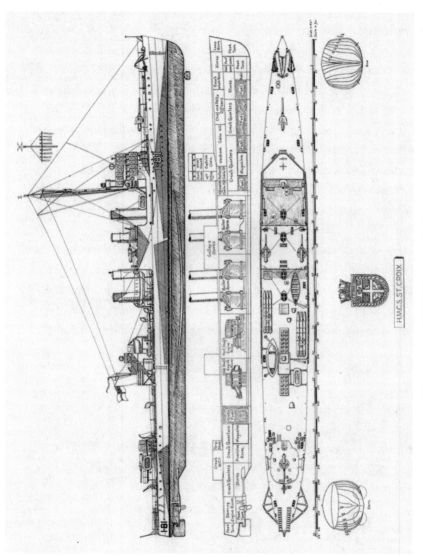

Line drawing of HMCS St. Croix, by L.B. Jenson.

Dobson, was awarded the Distinguished Service Cross for this success, but it wasn't gazetted until November 1942, long after *Ottawa* was gone.[84]

In 1938, the Royal Navy finally decided to start thinking seriously about a suitable design for an anti-submarine convoy escort vessel. A successful small whaling vessel called *Southern Pride* was adopted as the prototype and for a while was called a "Patrol Vessel, Whaler type." With his characteristic flair for tradition and history, Winston Churchill (when First Lord of the Admiralty in 1939) replaced this clumsy label with the name "corvette," the French for "sloop" in Napoleon's navy. Of course, it stuck. A corvette displaced 970 tons, could manage no more than sixteen knots, mounted a single four-inch gun of Great War vintage, an equally obsolete two-pounder twin Vickers pom-pom, and had a complement of forty-eight ratings and four officers. In 1940, these dumpy little ships had the bare minimum of anti-submarine weapons: four depth charge throwers and two depth charge rails at the stern. At first, their sole U-boat detection system was a very early Type 123A ASDIC. The little ship did, however, have one enormous tactical advantage over the much longer River class destroyer. It had a tighter turning circle than a submarine, which allowed it to easily outmanoeuvre a submerged or surfaced U-boat.

Corvettes could be built in non-Admiralty shipyards, when more sophisticated warships like destroyers could not. By the end of the war, 124 of these indomitable, rusty, cold, constantly wet, thoroughly uncomfortable, round-bottomed little ships had been built in various Canadian shipyards. It was said that they would "roll on wet grass," but nonetheless their sailors developed a sentimental attachment to them. All Royal Navy corvettes were named for flowers: *Gladiolus, Nasturtium, Hyacinth,* and *Pennywort,* for example. However, our naval chiefs in Ottawa preferred the names of Canadian towns to flowers: *Arvida, Barrie, Sherbrooke, Rosthern,* and *Chambly.*

In the summer of 1940, when the first corvettes were commissioned in both the Royal Navy and the Royal Canadian Navy, someone at the Admiralty decided that these ungainly little boats would best be commanded by RNR and RCNR officers, men with pre-war experience in merchant ships and ocean liners, and that their crews should come from the ranks of the volunteer reserve, men with little or no practical seagoing experience. Five of six escort ships in C-4 (*Ottawa* being the only exception) were commanded by ex-Merchant Marine RNR and RCNR officers. In 1941, the RCNR captain of a corvette was fortunate indeed if he discovered that just two or three of his senior ratings were experienced reservists out of a total ship's complement of forty-eight. The rest were green as grass and all too frequently had joined their newly commissioned little ships with a barely acceptable standard of training. But they had great spirit.

The short fo'c'sle and the open companionways characteristic of RCN corvettes meant that from the time that St. John's harbour was cleared until Londonderry was reached twelve to sixteen days later, everything you wore and everything around you was wet through. One naval veteran said that in order to appreciate life in a corvette, "you ought to go in to the bathroom on the coldest night of the year, open the window, fill the tub with water and then get in with your clothes on."[85] In spite of all these shortcomings, the corvette did her job magnificently. The sole survivor of the type, HMCS *Sackville*, is preserved as a national monument at dockside in Halifax, commemorating those who fought and won the Battle of the Atlantic in these little ships.

In 1939, the Royal Canadian Navy was really a tiny colonial clone of the Royal Navy. The Admiralty in London effectively controlled the destiny of the RCN: its orders came from Whitehall, its officers had been trained in Britain, and its ships were built there as well.

To proud Britons everywhere, the Royal Navy was the most powerful naval force in the world. The truly magnificent battle cruiser *Hood*, reputedly the largest warship afloat, showed the White Ensign to the delight of crowds in ports around the world during the twenties; the Royal Navy had huge warships with stirring names like *Courageous*, *Furious*, *Indomitable*, *Invincible*, and *Glorious*, dozens of cruisers, and hundreds of destroyers. In peacetime, all young professional RN officers (and, of course, RCN officers) were trained as either gunnery, torpedo, or signals specialists in addition to the standard naval education in navigation, engineering, and ship-handling.

In spite of the devastating effect that submarine warfare as conducted by the Imperial German Navy had had on the British people during the First World War, the professionals of the Royal Navy (and of its offspring, the Royal Canadian Navy) were surprisingly indifferent to the challenges of anti-submarine warfare. Accordingly, very few of either service's ships or men were equipped or prepared for it in September 1939.

The ten-year-old Royal Navy "C" and "D" class destroyers like *Crusader* (which became *Ottawa*) were designed in 1929 strictly for fleet escort work, surface gunnery action, and torpedo attacks. It did not seem to have occurred to the Admiralty that these ships would ever be used for anti-submarine warfare. In fact, on the eve of war in 1939, anti-submarine warfare was not considered a daunting challenge by Commodore (later Vice-Admiral) Percy Nelles, chief of the RCN's naval staff: "If international law is complied with, submarine attack should not prove serious. If unrestricted warfare is resorted to again [as it was in the Second World War], the means of combating submarines are considered to have so advanced, that by employing a system of convoy and utilizing air forces, losses of submarines would be very heavy and might compel the enemy to give up this form of attack."[86]

Percy Nelles was not alone in holding views like these. "It is interesting to reflect," Yogi Jenson wrote in his memoirs, that "despite the near strangling of Britain by German submarines in the Great War (1914–18), the subject of anti-submarine warfare was not touched upon in the lectures we [cadets] attended at the Royal Naval Tactical School in Portsmouth in 1938–9."[87]

Seagoing RCN officers (all trained with the Royal Navy in the U.K.) gave no more weight to the importance of anti-submarine warfare than did their own chief of naval staff. In September 1939, the RCN had only eight ratings trained in submarine detection and "two officers who had been on a course in anti-submarine warfare in 1927, but hadn't worked at it since."[88]

In September 1942, we tracked U-boats using ASDIC (or sonar, as the Americans called it), Radio Detection Finding (RDF, or radar), and HF/DF (High Frequency Direction Finding, or "Huff-Duff"). We destroyed them with depth charges, thrown or rolled off the stern of the ship.

ASDIC, the pioneer method of submarine detection, was invented in the last months of 1918, but the first equipment to be installed on ships was not designed until some years after the Great War. The Admiralty had suggested the acronym ASDIC from "Allied Submarine Detection Investigation Committee," a body that may or may not have been responsible for the invention and indeed may not have existed at all!

The principle of ASDIC was ingeniously simple: A sound transmitter housed in a dome mounted under the bottom of the ship sent out a narrow beam of high frequency sound. Using a simple hand wheel in the ship's radar hut near the bridge, an operator could direct the sonar beam. The beam gave off a characteristic *pinggggg* as it went out and an echo sound would return if the beam bounced off a solid object like a submarine (or a mine, a school of fish, or even a load of empty beer cans thrown overboard by the wardroom steward!). Water is an excellent conductor of sound, and the time difference between the beam and echo could very accurately estimate the distance to the submarine. The maximum range of this instrument was two thousand yards. Its only function was the detection of the presence, direction, and range of a fully submerged submarine.

When the war started, two of our original six destroyers did not even have ASDIC, and none of them had ever trained in submarine detection with a live submarine.[89]

On the other hand, RDF, or radar as it came to be called in 1943, could only detect objects projecting above the surface of the sea (or in the air), but it was of no use at all for the detection of submerged objects. In February 1935, Robert Watson-Watt, a brilliant Scottish physicist, produced a paper showing the possibility of using radio waves to detect the approach of aircraft in flight. In research done ten years earlier, he had calculated the height of the ionosphere above the earth's surface by measuring the interval between the emission of a radio pulse and the return of its echo, as recorded on a cathode-ray oscillograph. The next step was obvious. Two weeks after presenting his idea to a committee of his distinguished confreres, Watson-Watt was successfully bouncing radio waves off an RAF bomber in flight and radar was born. It has been stated on more than one occasion that radar and the famed Spitfire fighter aircraft won the Battle of Britain.

In March 1939, with war impending, the British government decided to share its greatest military secret with the Dominion governments. The Department of National Defence in Ottawa did not have a single physicist on its staff, but it did have a very close relationship with the National Research Council (NRC). Consequently, Ottawa chose Dr. John Henderson of the NRC to be Canada's representative for the secret meeting on radar held in London in April. Though Henderson was extensively briefed on the theoretical and practical aspects of the device and was shown through research centres and operational stations, he was bluntly informed that Dominion countries like Canada could expect nothing but basic technical information. It was up to each overseas dominion to develop technology to suit its own requirements and industrial practices.[90]

From this point on, the British government adopted an increasingly proprietary, secretive, and uncommunicative attitude in its dealings with the Canadians about radar. Indeed, the development of shipborne radar for Canadian warships was a muddle right from the start.[91] Percy Nelles, the chief of the naval staff, cherished a dream that RCN destroyers would become part of a great imperial fleet directed entirely from the Admiralty in London. When, in 1939, this was abruptly shattered by Prime Minister William Lyon Mackenzie King's insistence on autonomy for Canada's navy, the Admiralty decided that the Canadians could fend for themselves "when it came to finding the equipment necessary for its warships," including the development of radar technology.[92] From then on, there was a yawning gap between British and Canadian radar development.

Following the fall of France and the vast expansion of U-boat warfare made possible by the establishment of submarine bases in the Biscay ports (Brest, La Rochelle, and Lorient), the Royal Canadian Navy became increasingly involved in protecting convoys from submarine attack in the middle and western Atlantic. We used ten-year-old destroyers that were never intended to seek out and sink submarines and brand new corvettes purposely designed for this job.

In February 1940, a group of scientists at Birmingham designed the cavity magnetron valve, which enabled the development of the far more accurate shortwave radar. The valve allowed the transmission of much stronger radio signals, thereby increasing the power available in the centimetric range by a thousand-fold. Tests done by HMS *Orchis* in May 1941 demonstrated the ability of the new 271 prototype, with its cavity magnetron technology, to detect with ease a "trimmed down" submarine (meaning with only its conning tower appearing above the surface) up to a distance of thirty-five hundred yards at night. This revolutionized anti-submarine warfare, and the U-boat was soon to be robbed of its most effective tactic.

Naval Service Headquarters (NSHQ) realized full well that the RCN had no scientific research development capability of its own. Furthermore, in responding to the Admiralty's urgent appeals for technical help in 1940, the RCN had been virtually picked clean of its few trained radar officers and technicians.[93]

NSHQ had also become uncomfortably aware that there was no scientific liaison between the RCN and the Admiralty on the British development of advanced shortwave centimetric radar. Accordingly, in January 1941, the NRC was designated as the official scientific research establishment for the navy. At that point, Canadian naval liaison in London was woefully understaffed, with one staff officer (material) who looked after everything from ship engines to radar. It seemed a puzzling decision, therefore, that C.J. Mackenzie, the president of NRC, decided against establishing a liaison office in London. Thus, there was no meaningful contact between the British scientific establishment and the NRC or the RCN on the advances in radar development that were already proceeding very quickly indeed in the United Kingdom. The British were reluctant to share their research data with Canada: they would wait until their new centimetric radar set was in production before they would provide any related technical information. As a result, the RCN and the NRC would remain significantly behind the Admiralty in radar development for much of the war. Because of both

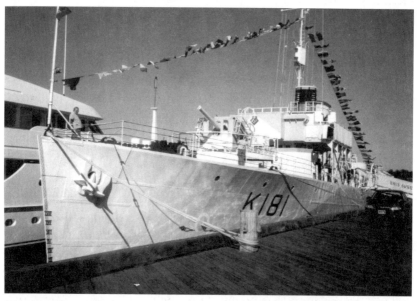

The characteristic "lantern" of the Type 271 radar perched atop the radar hut just abaft the bridge of HMCS Sackville, *the last surviving Second World War corvette, lovingly preserved at dockside in Halifax Harbour. This Perspex shield protected the sensitive dipole aerials from the elements. (Courtesy of Dr. James Goodwin.)*

the NRC's failure to establish an effective scientific and technical liaison overseas with the Admiralty and continuing British insensitivity, NSHQ would be completely unaware of the existence of Type 271 centimetric radar until June 1941.[94]

Before the war, the Royal Navy had focused on radar for anti-aircraft and gunnery control sets on major warships. When the need for surface scanning radar became important, the navy acquired compact air-to-surface

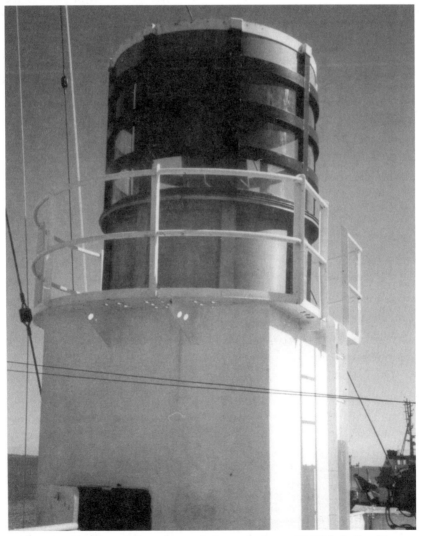

A close-up of the trademark "lantern" atop the 271 radar hut on HMCS Sackville. *(Courtesy of Dr. James Goodwin.)*

vessel sets from the RAF, which could be fitted on destroyers and came to be called Type 286. Almost immediately, however, this set had obvious limitations. Operating on a wavelength of 1.5 metres, it lacked the discrimination necessary to detect a submarine's echo in rough seas. Their antennas had serious weaknesses. They could not be rotated and could only scan in a forward arc. Accordingly, the whole ship had to be turned towards the contact in order to get an accurate bearing.[95]

By January 1941, all seven RCN destroyers had been fitted with the long-wave (1.5-metre) 286M radar in Britain. Soon after this, at the navy's request, the NRC began working on a Canadian prototype, the Canadian Sea Control set. This was to be the basis for a production model called SW1C, or Surface Warning One Canadian. It quickly became known as "Swick."

The first sea trials of Swick were conducted by HMCS *Chambly* (whose captain was the legendary Commander J.D. "Chummy" Prentice, RCN) in May 1941 and were deemed very successful. The set could accurately detect a fully surfaced test submarine in clear weather. The ruinous defect of both the 286M radar and Swick was that they could not detect a submarine approaching when it was trimmed down. As this was the standard practice of German U-boats during night attacks in the Battle of the Atlantic, it effectively rendered the 286M and Swick radar sets useless.

At the same time that HMCS *Chambly* was announcing the success of Swick, the RN corvette HMS *Orchis* was testing the completely new Type 271 centimetric radar set, with outstanding results. It is a sad fact that no Canadian escort warship in the summer of 1942 had Type 271 radar equipment. This was to have tragic consequences for *Ottawa*, 114 of her men, and 22 merchant seamen (rescued by *Ottawa*) from the torpedoed *Empire Oil.*

By early January 1942, seventy-eight British escort warships were already fitted with Type 271 radar when the RCN had just begun to equip its vessels with the increasingly faulty 1.5-metre sets.[96] Once again, because of poor liaison and British insensitivity, the RCN was left completely in the dark. Swick radar had failed miserably. There was only one instance in which it detected a submarine approaching on the surface. This was in August 1942, when HMCS *Sackville* detected two U-boats, but because of the radar's limited range, both escaped. A senior British officer remarked cuttingly that a ship fitted with a Type 271 centimetric set would have found both targets a gift.[97]

There is little doubt that RCN convoy disasters in the fall of 1942, particularly the one that befell ON 127 in September, were contributed to in no small degree by the procrastination of the naval staff in Ottawa in planning for a centimetric radar fitting and supply policy. Indeed, discussions on this urgent initiative dragged on from March 2 to October 1, 1942, and "this doomed RCN escorts always to remain behind in the mounting of the latest electronic hardware."[98]

Early in these discussions, the fitting of centimetric radar (Type 271 and the Canadian version, the RX/C) hit a snag. Admiral Nelles and the naval staff saw that fitting the new centimetric radar equipment would require removal of central gunnery directory control equipment and the optical gear carried for range-finding. There just wasn't enough room for both behind the bridge of a River class destroyer. There were still some senior naval officers at NSHQ who clung to the traditional view that the only proper function of the destroyer was in a fleet support role, and this demanded the preservation of the directory control of the ship's guns.

In a memorandum (98423) marked "Secret" and dated July 29, 1942, the commanding officer of *Ottawa*, Lieutenant Commander C.A. Rutherford, summarized his observations on the status of the ship's 286M radar equipment as follows: "This set although when working, produces results compatible with the expected performance, is completely obsolete. It has been arranged to acquire the necessary equipment on the next occasion of ship's visit to Londonderry for the conversion of this set.... It is hoped that this modification may be carried out at this time."

This memo was duly received on August 13, 1942, by the Captain (D) Newfoundland, Captain E.R. Mainguy, RCN, and by the Flag Officer Newfoundland Force, Rear Admiral L.W. Murray, RCN, who both concurred in Rutherford's conclusion that the set was "completely obsolete."

On August 4, 1942, before he had received the above memorandum, Captain Mainguy had requested permission to have the River class destroyers *Skeena* and *Saguenay* fitted with Type 271 radar in Londonderry. However, the NSHQ brass couldn't make up their minds and deferred to Their Lordships of the Admiralty in London, who delayed their advice until October, by which time *Ottawa* had been lost.

This indecision by the naval staff over the displacement of the traditional range-finding gear by the new Type 271 radar fitting seems to have made its way down to *Ottawa*'s captain, Lieutenant Commander Rutherford, as her young gunnery officer, Sub-Lieutenant Yogi Jenson found to his dismay:

> The final time we were alongside in Londonderry, I ... was informed by the dockyard authorities that we were to be fitted with an RDF 271 in lieu of the [main gunnery] rangefinder [atop the bridge]. The 271 arrived alongside ... and I casually informed the captain, who I assumed had been informed about this. He became very upset and seemed to have the impression that I had authorized this on my own. I was to cancel it at once, which I did. I was very sorry as I was ... very aware of the limitations of the 286M RDF [Radar].[99]

He (and indeed everyone else in *Ottawa*) was to regret this in twelve days' time.

Compounding this tragic shambles was the fact that *Celandine*, the RN corvette, was the only ship in C-4 escort group with Type 271 radar, but it was unserviceable at a critical time in the next week.

In August 1942, the *Kriegsmarine* came up with an electronic device that effectively disabled the already flawed Canadian anti-submarine tracking capability. German engineers designed a radar search receiver, the *Funkmesserbeobachtung* (FuMB), or Metox, that could detect long-wave (metric) radar emissions from the 286 and SW1C sets fitted on nearly all Canadian escorts but was unable to pick up the shortwave (centimetric) emissions from 271 radar. This probably explains, at least in part, the failure of RCN ships to sink more than a very small number of U-boats in the fall of 1942 and into the spring of 1943.

There was another grave deficiency in our ability to protect convoys. Five hundred miles west of Northern Ireland and the same distance east of Newfoundland, there was a huge area in the middle of the North Atlantic with no air cover at all. This was the infamous "Black Pit." Until we had very long range aircraft like the Liberator and some of the new escort aircraft carriers to close this gap, the U-boat wolf packs could continue to attack with impunity. Convoy ON 127 reached the eastern rim of the Black Pit on September 9.

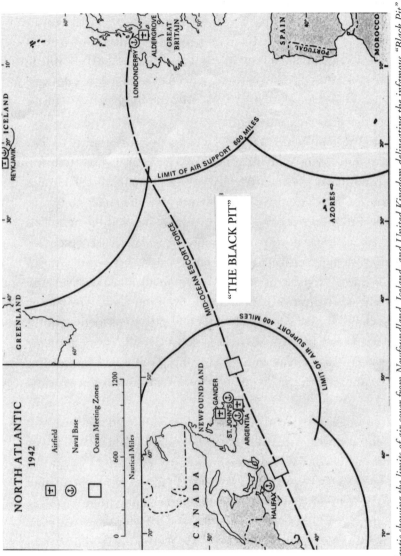

Map of the North Atlantic showing the limits of air cover from Newfoundland, Iceland, and United Kingdom delineating the infamous "Black Pit" through which a convoy had to pass without any protection from the air. (Adapted from map on page 238 of At War At Sea: Sailors and Naval Combat in the 20th Century by Ronald H. Spector, copyright © 2001 by Ronald H. Spector. Used by permission of Viking Penguin, a division of Penguin Group [USA] Inc.)

It is a fact of naval history that the protection afforded by the convoy system was demonstrated several centuries ago. It unquestionably saved ships, cargo, and men. However, it took the eruption of unrestricted submarine warfare by the Imperial German Navy in February 1917, with its appalling ship slaughter, to finally convince Admiral Sir John Jellicoe (he of Jutland fame) and Their Lordships of the Admiralty that hurried establishment of the convoy system was the vital tactic that would save Britain from starvation. With the implementation of convoys, ship losses dropped dramatically. The U-boat could no longer destroy independent ships by surface gunfire, boarding, and scuttling.

A typical Second World War convoy was composed of thirty to sixty merchant ships carrying everything from raw materials (wheat, iron ore, cotton) to oil, tanks, locomotives, planes, and ammunition. The ships were organized into nine to twelve columns one thousand yards (five cables) apart, each one spaced five hundred yards ahead of the next. This produced a huge rectangle, five times or more as wide as it was deep. This arrangement was quite deliberate. As merchant ships presented the biggest target from bow to stern, each column was kept to no more than five ships, thus reducing the threat of U-boat attack from the flank. The convoy would be commanded by a retired senior RN officer, referred to as the commodore, whose chief task was to keep slow older ships from straggling and to keep civilian captains in line. The ships in so-called fast convoys could manage nine to fifteen knots and those in slow convoys between six and nine knots.

Each convoy had an identifying code name. Eastbound convoys to the United Kingdom were prefixed with the letters *HX* (Halifax to U.K.) or *SC* (Sydney to U.K.). Westbound convoys were prefixed *ON* (U.K. to Halifax) or *ONS* (U.K. to Halifax slow). ON 127 was a fast westbound convoy in ballast and it was in two sections, one sailing from the Clyde and the other from Loch Ewe, a remote anchorage high on the west coast of Scotland, which served as an assembly point for those ships routed from east coast British ports around the northern tip of the Scottish mainland through the Pentland Firth and down the Minch into the Loch. These ships were so routed to avoid the obvious risk of passage through the Strait of Dover and the Western English Channel.

The rendezvous of the Clyde section of the convoy with *St. Croix,*

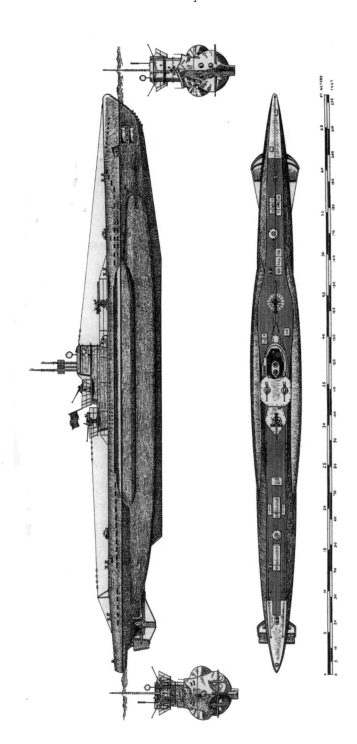

Line drawing of U-91, the Type VIIC German submarine that sank HMCS Ottawa, by L.B. Jenson.

Ottawa, and the four corvettes of Escort Group C-4 took place uneventfully at 1135 BST (British Summer Time). The Loch Ewe section joined at 1845, and Convoy ON 127 set a course of 262° homeward bound into the North Atlantic.

The Type VIIC submarine was the mainstay of the German navy throughout the war. These 769-ton boats were marvels of compactness. Within their 220-foot-long pressure hull, they had to accommodate forty-four men (including four officers), enough food for sixty days and sometimes longer, four torpedo tubes forward and one aft, storage space for twenty torpedoes, and a great mass of pipes, valves, cables, and other control machinery. Two powerful diesel engines could drive a boat at a top speed of eighteen knots on the surface, and the paired electric motors could propel it at a maximum of four to seven knots when submerged. The diesels did double duty on the surface by charging the huge seven-ton batteries for the electric motors.

The theory and practice of the wolf-pack attack, or *rudeltaktik*, was the inspired conception of Grosadmiral Karl Dönitz, the commander-in-chief of the German U-boat Service, or *Befehlshaber der Unterseebooten* (BdU). He had conceived this innovation in tactics from his experience as a U-boat commander in the Great War and conducted a very successful mock convoy killing exercise in the Baltic Sea well before the war in 1938.

By the end of August 1942, there were in excess of one hundred U-boats loose in the Atlantic, and twenty-four of these were marshalled into three wolf packs, called *Lohs* (nine boats), *Stier* (six boats), and *Vorwärts* (nine boats). Dönitz's attack plan called for the pack to spread out into a gigantic vertical net across the path of the oncoming convoy with individual boats three miles apart. When one member of the pack sighted the convoy, this report was sent by wireless to BdU headquarters in Kerneval, a small town on the Biscay coast of France just north of Lorient, and orders were then relayed to the others to converge for the attack. Convoy position and U-boat orders were determined on a plot of the entire Atlantic Ocean (North and South), the Caribbean, the Mediterranean Sea, and even around the Cape of Good Hope into the Indian Ocean. Keyed to conventional longitude and latitude, it consisted of a series of large lettered grid squares containing a host of much smaller numbered squares, and these were labelled accordingly (thus, "BD 61" corresponded to 42°

W 47° N). This was an exclusively German innovation[100]: the RN and the RCN used conventional longitude-latitude navigational reckoning throughout the war.

Using these simple coordinates, the U-boats would then be directed to attack their prey at night and on the surface, literally ambushing the convoy. They would run in head on for as long as they could and would submerge only if discovered or in preparation for the final attack. A submarine was nine or ten knots faster on the surface than when submerged, and this was a decided advantage during night attacks. ASDIC was of no use for detecting the U-boat on the surface. Only high-precision radar like the Type 271 could do that, but, regrettably, no Canadian ship had this equipment installed until late in 1942. Because the Germans continued to communicate recklessly using wireless radio transmission, HF/DF could track them when transmitting on the surface, but once again none of our ships were equipped with this equipment until much later.

However, it wasn't all roses for the wolf packs. They were vulnerable, too. The farther west they were sent, the greater their supply problems and the shorter the time available for attacks. Occasionally, they could rendezvous with a big *milchcow* boat bringing the indispensable fuel, food, and torpedoes. Hunting convoys in the terrible North Atlantic winter weather could be frustratingly difficult. If a wolf pack numbered twenty or twenty-five U-boats, patrol lines could stretch out to well over one hundred miles. When the call discovering a convoy went out from a boat at one end of the line, it might be impossible for the rest of the pack to close in on the convoy in time and the attack might be a failure. It was after one such failure (an abortive attack on convoy SC 97 in late August) that Dönitz ordered thirteen boats to form a reinforced *Vorwärts* ("Forward") wolf pack: U-92, U-584, U-659, U-96, U-404, U-608, U-594, U-218, U-380, U-211, U-407, U-411, and U-91.

U-91 was brand new. She had been built in Lübeck on the Baltic Sea and was commissioned in January 1942. This was her first patrol. Her captain was twenty-seven-year-old Oberleutnant zur See Heinz Walkerling, who took command with but fifteen months' experience in submarines.

U-91 had sailed from Kiel on August 15, 1942, and joined the *Vorwärts* group that had been thrown out into a very long north–south patrol line on the eastern rim of the notorious Black Pit, like a huge net with its boats deployed miles apart ready to pounce on the oncoming convoy ON 127.

At 2100 of September 9, 1942, U-584 at the southern end of the net made the first sighting of the ships of ON 127, lost them, and then found them again the next day. This was now assuming the proportions of an ambush as five of her wolf pack mates made contact with the hapless convoy. One of them, U-96, was soon like a fox among the chickens. She managed to hit three ships in rapid succession at 1431z. Two ships, *Sveve* and *Elisabeth Van Belgie*, were so badly damaged in the attack that *Sherbrooke* was ordered to sink them both by gunfire, after rescuing their crews. The third ship, *F.J. Wolfe*, managed to limp along under its own power and ultimately made it into St. John's on September 18.

The other escorts now swung into action. *St. Croix*, *Ottawa*, *Arvida*, and *Celandine* began sweeps. Three attacking boats (U-594, U-404, and U-584) were driven deep by depth charges from *Arvida* and *St. Croix*. Later, *Ottawa* was ordered to a position well astern of ON 127 in order to prevent a submarine from surfacing and shadowing the convoy.

At 1715z, U-659 torpedoed the tanker *Empire Oil* and then was driven off by *St. Croix*. All but two of the tanker's crew of fifty-one were rescued, twenty-six by *St. Croix* and twenty-three by *Ottawa*, including a badly injured DEMS gunner who would be operated on the next day.[101] When the badly damaged ship slipped astern of the convoy, she was finished off by U-584. At 2225z, three more freighters were torpedoed by U-218, U-404, and U-608. *Marit II* and *Fjordaas* managed to keep up with the convoy in spite their damage, but *Liberty Glo* was not seen again.

A series of ASDIC contacts up to 0200z was made by *Arvida*, *Amherst*, and *Ottawa*, but only *Arvida's* depth charge attack seemed to have produced any significant damage. By daylight on September 11, the radar equipment on all the escorts had failed, including *Celandine's* superior Type 271 set. Eight more U-boats chose this moment to swoop down on ON 127. At 1723z, *Hindanger* was torpedoed by U-584 and was later sunk as a derelict by *Amherst*. Then at 2300z, U-211 slipped in easily under the screen and torpedoed both *Hektoria* and *Empire Moonbeam*. Both these ships were sunk later by U-608.

September 12 passed quietly but the preceding forty-eight hours had seen seven ships sunk, another five able to carry on in spite of damage, and one simply vanish.

However, in spite of the inaccuracy of the escort warship depth charge attacks, U-boat commanders had to be pretty nimble to escape. When U-boats submerged to 150 to 160 metres, they were slowed right down to four knots or even less and were thus effectively out of action. Now, on the morning of September 13, they were rapidly approaching the western edge of the Black Pit and could expect the devastating attack of long-range bomber aircraft out of Newfoundland.

For *Gruppe Vorwärts*, the time of the easy kill was nearly at an end.

DOCTOR IN HIS CABIN OPERATING ROOM HERO OF PLUNGING OTTAWA

Hadn't Strength Left After Four Sleepless Days to Save Own Life

DYING MEN SANG

By ERIC HUTTON

An Eastern Canadian Port, Sept. 26—Two major operations performed aboard a plunging destroyer at sea, followed by four days and nights without sleep, attending to his patients, cost the life of Surgeon-Lieut. George Hendry of Toronto, medical officer aboard H.M.C.S. Ottawa. The Ottawa was torpedoed in the battle of the Atlantic with a loss of two-thirds of her crew.

"If I had to name a hero of that battle we had out there," said Lieut. Dunn Lantier, of Montreal, rescued officer of the Ottawa, "I would put Dr. Hendry alongside our commander, Larry Rutherford. Both of them had been without sleep for four days and nights before we were torpedoed—Larry commanding his ship in a running battle with subs, and Hendry working like a Trojan on two cases he would have been lucky to save if he had had a city hospital's facilities at his disposal.

"When the time came to save themselves, there in the water hanging on to rafts, they just had nothing left. They slipped away before the rescue vessels could reach us."

Operated on Survivor

Lieut. Lantier, who left his post as aide-de-camp to Canada's governor-general to join the navy, was interviewed aboard the ship which brought him, together with three other officers of the Ottawa and some 50 ratings, to this port

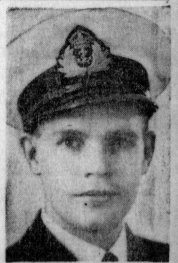

SURGEON-LIEUT. HENDRY

from the base to which the rescue vessels took them after picking up survivors "somewhere in the Atlantic."

"The men of the Ottawa just about worshipped Dr. Hendry," he said. "He was their sports officer and one of the most popular men on board. The survivors feel his loss terribly.

"The first man he operated on was a merchant seaman we had picked up after his ship was torpedoed. An iron bolt had been blown into his stomach by the explosion. All Dr. Hendry had for a 'hospital' was a small cabin. He operated on that seaman twice, and the first time the patient had to be lashed to the table to keep him in place, the seas were running so high, and it was all the rest of us could do to keep our footing. Later,

(Continued on page 3, col. 3)

The Toronto Daily Star *for September 26, 1942, gave details of George Hendry's magnificent surgical performance and his death. In keeping with strict wartime censorship, this was sent in from "An Eastern Canadian Port," which was St. John's, Newfoundland, where* Ottawa*'s survivors were brought.*

"Doctor in His Cabin
Operating Room
Hero of Plunging Ottawa"[102]

*N*ow we have to turn the clock back to Sunday, September 6, 1942, the day after *Ottawa* sailed from Lough Foyle to join the convoy in the North Channel off Rathlin Island. At 0830 that morning, Able Seaman William "Pooch" Bucheski of Windsor, Ontario, reported to the sickbay with severe abdominal pain, loss of appetite, nausea, and vomiting. After examination, Dr. Hendry made the only possible diagnosis: acute appendicitis. He then went directly to the captain and told him that Bucheski would have to be operated on within forty-eight hours. It all boiled down to one of two equally difficult choices: either turn the ship around and return the man to port for operation, thus seriously weakening the convoy's protection, or perform the surgery on board. To deplete the escort force to that extent was clearly impossible, so Hendry agreed to go ahead.

T.C. Pullen recalls, "'Pooch' Bucheski, our patient, a popular member of the ship's company, will always be remembered for a particular reason. During one of our boisterous hockey games in Halifax, Seamen versus the Wardroom, he unintentionally, so I like to think, clipped me in the mouth with his stick. The dead tooth that resulted has lasted to this day, a constant reminder of far-off days of yore and gore."[103]

In the course of the next five days, in the cramped captain's day cabin of a small warship in mid-Atlantic, George Hendry would carry out two major surgical operations, the second far more complicated than the first, while the convoy and its escorts (including *Ottawa*) were being ambushed by a wolf pack of thirteen U-boats. This remarkable performance was never equalled anywhere during the Second World War.

In 1942, Surgeon Lieutenant Commander Walter MacKenzie set the scene very well when he referred to "medical officers serving at sea and having the sole responsibility for their ship's complement. This assignment may entail long periods with a small body of normally healthy men, and one may feel that his professional knowledge is not being adequately utilized. Suddenly, without warning, disaster is upon them and the medical officer has every opportunity to test his ability and ingenuity. He is on his own, without the service of a consultant."[104]

An RCN document entitled "Medical Organization in Destroyers" advises that "the scope of the surgeon's activities will be measured to some extent by the type of ship in which he is serving. For example, the medical officer in a small ship can perform relatively little surgery compared to that possible in a battleship or battle-cruiser carrying three or more medical officers and a half-a-dozen sick berth staff."[105] Destroyers normally carried one medical officer and one sick berth attendant. In *Ottawa*, Leading Sick Berth Attendant Alexander MacMillan

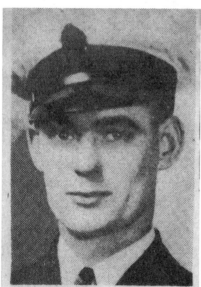

MISSING IN OTTAWA ACTION
Alexander MacMillan, Kingston, sick bay attendant aboard the lost Canadian destroyer Ottawa, who aided Surgeon Lieut. George Hendry in caring for the wounded aboard the vessel. He is listed as missing.

"Missing in Ottawa *action": Leading Sick Berth Attendant Alexander MacMillan, who assisted Surgeon Lieutenant George Hendry at two major operations on board HMCS* Ottawa *and was lost when the ship was torpedoed in mid-Atlantic. (Toronto Daily Star, September 26, 1942.)*

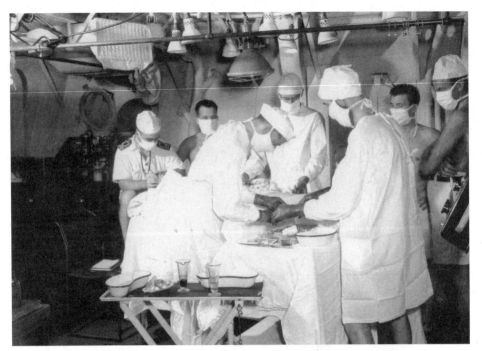

Appendicitis surgery on board the eight-thousand-ton cruiser HMCS Uganda, *August 1945. (Courtesy of W.G.P. Rawling, from* Death Their Enemy *[Ottawa: privately published, 2001].)*

was the other member of what T.C. Pullen referred to as "our two-man medical team."[106]

Even in 1942, the removal of an inflamed appendix dangling from its typical attachment to the base of the caecum (that segment of the large bowel lying in the right lower quadrant of the abdominal cavity) was usually a pretty straightforward procedure, if it was done in a good-sized city hospital with ample help from trained professionals. Approaching the appendix through a short, six- to seven-centimetre oblique incision, the surgeon would separate muscle, open the peritoneum (the "skin" lining the abdominal cavity) to expose the underlying appendix, free it from its mooring mesentery, clamp it across its base, and finally remove it by transection with a scalpel. The sutured stump would be treated with iodine and the site checked carefully for oozing blood loss. Finally the peritoneum, muscle layers, subcutaneous fat, and skin would be brought together and closed with catgut and silk sutures. An experienced surgeon could have this done in little more time than it takes to describe it, frequently in twenty to twenty-five minutes.

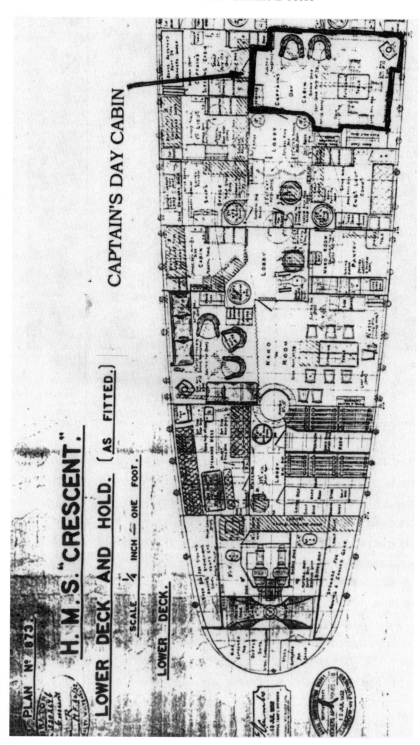

CAPTAIN'S DAY CABIN

Admiralty Plan # 873 (dated July 12, 1932) for the stern half of the lower deck for HMS Crescent (to become HMCS Fraser), the common prototype for HMS Crusader (to become HMCS Ottawa), HMS Comet (to become HMCS Restigouche), and HMS Cygnet (to become HMCS St. Laurent). Outlined is the location of the captain's day cabin. (Courtesy of Captain W.M. Caswell, MVO, Royal Navy, and the former shipbuilder, Vickers-Armstrong, Ltd., Barrow-in-Furness, U.K.)

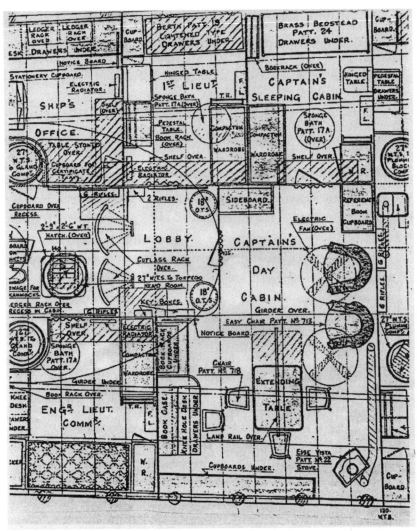

An enlargement of the lower deck plan (opposite) shows details of the captain's day cabin where two major surgical operations were carried out. The space available for these procedures was just 16 x 10–12 feet. Because of the ship's rolling, each patient had to be tied down on the small dining table in the centre of the cabin. Note "cutlass racks" in this post-Nelson warship (dead centre of the plan)!

When he agreed to carry out these procedures on board *Ottawa*, George Hendry told the captain, Lieutenant Commander Larry Rutherford, that he would need a lot of help. A suitable site had to be found for conversion into a makeshift operating room. In larger warships this was no problem, but as the sick bay in a "C" class destroyer was little bigger than a closet, at seven feet by ten feet, they had to settle on the captain's day cabin located on the lower deck aft.[107] The available space measured sixteen by twelve feet, and the cabin was furnished with an extending dining table very suitable for the proposed operation.

When his anticipated leave home to Toronto (to prepare for his divorce petition hearing) in mid-December 1941 was frustrated by the Japanese attack on Pearl Harbor and he was finally posted to Halifax for sea duty, George Hendry predicted (accurately as it turned out) that he might have to do emergency abdominal surgery afloat. He wanted to be ready for it. After all, he'd had considerably more postgraduate surgical training than the average medical officer in these small warships, and, according to Yogi Jenson, this was certainly true of George's predecessor. Whether they did surgery in small ships or small towns, the average Canadian medical graduate in the 1930s and 1940s had to be resourceful and self-reliant, and Hendry was no exception. When he joined *Ottawa* in Halifax Dockyard, he did a rapid inventory of the ship's skimpy sick bay and found it decidedly wanting. The various lists of contents for medical chests and first aid lockers, promulgated in Admiralty Fleet Orders (AFOs), contained little more than those instruments necessary for suturing lacerations — certainly far short of those required for major surgery, inhalation anaesthetics, and intravenous administration of saline or transfused blood.

The only surviving Admiralty documents listing the contents of medical chests or sick bay lockers include very few instruments, drugs, or related materials that would be useful during major surgery at sea. They contained (among other items):

- anaesthetics, not specified
- goose neck lamp
- ligatures, not specified
- artery forceps
- scissors

- dressing forceps
- scalpel
- glass hypodermic syringes
- dried blood serum
- syrettes
- morphine[108]

"Surgical instruments" included:

- peritoneum forceps
- dissecting forceps
- Mayo-Oschner forceps
- syringes – 10 mL
- needles for syringes, size not specified[109]

So it was clear that George Hendry would have to acquire the equipment, instruments, drugs, and other materials for the surgery he had in mind by applying for it (or by scrounging whatever he felt was necessary) from the RCN Hospital at *Stadacona*. In fact, AFO 2530, dated July 4, 1940, expressly advises this course of action: "Medical officers are to apply to their appropriate storing hospital [in this case, RCNH Halifax] for such articles."

In 1942, the following would have been the bare minimum of the contemporary equipment required even for a routine procedure like an appendectomy:

- surgical instruments:
  - scalpels, one piece (would need sharpening after each use)
  - Kocher forceps
  - arterial forceps ("snaps")
  - surgical scissors ("Metzenbaum")
  - thumb forceps
  - needle holder or "driver"
  - free needles (like sewing needles; no "swaged-on" needles then)
  - small "ribbon" retractors (there were probably none larger)
- suture material (probably packaged in spools):
  - catgut: chromic, size 00, 0, and # 1

> - silk: size 00, 0, and # 1
- rubber gloves
- gauze bandages, a large supply, fashioned into what were (and still are) called "sponges," to make up for the lack of surgical suction, an essential bit of equipment for emergency abdominal surgery
- ether plus gauze mask for administration
- intravenous tubing: stainless steel connectors
- needles, stainless steel: # 22, 20, 18
- glass syringes: hypodermic, 5 mL, 10 mL, 20 mL, and 50 mL
- rubber tubing: to serve as nasogastric tube
- catheter: simple and/or retention type
- sterilizer(s)
- towels to "drape" the OR field
- cotton masks, perhaps plus OR caps and gowns, if they could be found
- alcohol and iodine: antiseptics for preparing the skin preoperatively

In those days, there were no disposable items. Everything had to be cleaned, sterilized, and reused: instruments, syringes, needles, gloves, tubing, towels — everything.

Other than Leading Sick Berth Attendant Alexander MacMillan, no member of the ship's crew had training or experience with medical care of any kind, and as he would need an assistant or two during the operation, Dr. Hendry had to take on novice helpers and give them some very rapid practical instruction.

Hendry had nothing more sophisticated than ether anaesthesia to rely on, and he had to give MacMillan a lightning brush-up on the essentials of its administration, maintenance, and monitoring.

As anaesthesia was, at that time, an infant clinical specialty without much sophistication, it seems reasonable to assume that ether would have been used, being the most commonly employed agent. It was safe, it was not as toxic as chloroform or cyclopropane, and it wouldn't get the occasional anaesthetist into trouble.

George Hendry probably induced (started) the anaesthetic himself but then passed it to SBA MacMillan for continued administration, maintenance, and monitoring while he got on with the surgery.

The technique of simple inhalation anaesthesia involved the dropping of ether directly from the bottle that it was supplied in onto a gauze mask secured on a wire frame and applied gently to the patient's face. There are four classical stages of anaesthesia: the stages of conscious inhalation and excitement are involved with the induction of the anaesthetic; the third stage of deep anaesthesia is concerned with its maintenance; and the last stage is recovery. Surgical anaesthesia has been attained when there is muscular relaxation with total absence of pain and quiet, uniform breathing. As the anaesthetist, SBA MacMillan would have to monitor the patient repeatedly to make sure that his pulse was slow, respirations regular, pupils constricted, and skin pink. Only a little ether was required to maintain a satisfactory level of anaesthesia, but once this had been achieved, MacMillan would have to keep the drop rate absolutely constant. It was a very practical axiom that uneven administration of ether anaesthetic resulted in uneven anaesthesia.

Monday, September 7, 1942

Everything was in readiness in the captain's day cabin, including a couple of very serviceable operating room lights that had been manufactured and rigged by Mr. Lloyd Jones, the torpedo gunner, and W.H. Hobbis, the electrical artificer. The operation "was performed during the afternoon in a moderate sea and with considerable motion on the ship.... Bucheski had to be lashed to the dining table and braced firmly by his shipmates against the rolling and the pitching."[110] Though he couldn't recall almost half a century later why Bob Billard, *Ottawa's* shipwright (the ship's carpenter), was recruited as an operating room helper, Tom Pullen thought it was "perhaps because he was handy with tools (albeit of a cruder sort) ... somehow he might come in useful."

Once Doc got down to the bloody business of cut and thrust, there were defections from the ranks of the amateur helpers. Tom Pullen, "no longer an observer, became instead a fetcher and carrier until the job was done. Three hours it lasted," but this hardly comes as a surprise. Bucheski was a big man, and even under the best conditions, big people can be difficult to operate on and to anaesthetize. With the ship rolling around in a rough sea, Alex

MacMillan was probably having his hands full trying to maintain a satisfactory level of anaesthesia and to keep the big guy from retching. Add to that the possibility that the appendix might have been tucked way in behind the bowel that it's attached to (the so-called retrocaecal appendix), which can make it difficult to remove, and three hours is not at all unusual.

The appendectomy George Hendry did on board HMCS *Ottawa* was the first of three such procedures carried out at sea on the North Atlantic during the Second World War. Because these operations were performed sixty years ago and were necessarily cloaked in security restrictions, the recorded descriptions of the second and third appendectomies are sketchy, anecdotal, and incomplete.

It was when HMCS *Haida*, one of the new (and much larger) Tribal class destroyers, was escorting a returning Murmansk convoy in November of 1943 that one of her young ratings, fearful of the surgical attentions of the Russian doctors in that cold and forbidding port, delayed reporting his suggestive abdominal pain and nausea until *Haida* was well out to sea and not likely to return to Murmansk. By that time, his appendicitis was advanced, and rapid preparations were made for the necessary procedure. The medical officer, Surgeon Lieutenant Commander Samuel A. MacDonald, then performed the operation with the sick berth attendant acting as both first assistant and scrub nurse. The ship's writer and her paymaster acted as willing "gofers," and her legendary captain, Commander Harry DeWolf, kept the ship on as even a keel as possible. The patient made a full recovery.[111]

The third appendectomy was carried out "somewhere in the Atlantic" on a Royal Navy destroyer (unnamed in the press release from "An Eastern Canadian Port" for security reasons) on July 6, 1944, by twenty-nine-year-old Surgeon Lieutenant Bruce A. Campbell, RCNVR, of Strathroy, Ontario.[112] Both the patient, Able Seaman A.H. King, and the anaesthetist, Surgeon Lieutenant Budd (both of the Royal Naval Volunteer Reserve), had to be transferred by ship's boat from their RN corvette on a fortunately calm sea.

"The captain's day cabin was converted into a little operating theatre, the dining table served as an operating table, sterilizers were placed on the writing desk, instruments were laid out ready for action as neatly as in any well appointed hospital and lighting of sufficient power was rigged in quick time by the Torpedo Gunner."[113] Surgeon Lieutenant Campbell "went to work with scalpel and suture," assisted by the first lieutenant, who had "seen some operations, but had never been so close. Using a white cap-cover and a handkerchief to form a makeshift mask, Dr. Campbell dealt effectively with an appendix so recalcitrant that the job finally took an hour and a half."

These were by no means the only appendectomies performed afloat during the war.[114] Far away in the Pacific Theatre, just a few days after George Hendry had operated on Pooch Bucheski in the middle of the North Atlantic, Pharmacist's Mate First Class Wheeler B. Lipes removed the appendix of a seaman named Darrel Rector on board the American submarine USS *Seadragon*. The decidedly enterprising Lipes used a tea strainer lined with gauze as an ether mask and bent tablespoons from the sub's galley as retractors. The patient recovered. Then, in 1943, a navy corpsman named Thomas A. Moore on board another submarine, USS *Silversides*, took out another appendix under similar circumstances and with similar results. This time, the brass of the USN Medical Corps forbade the future performance of appendectomy by other than qualified physicians. Notwithstanding this edict, yet another "submarine appendectomy" was carried out by PhM 1C Harry Roby on USS *Grayback* later in 1943!

Next for George Hendry came a surgical challenge that made an appendectomy seem like a walk in the park, even though it had been done on the high seas in a little cabin on a small warship.

Tuesday, September 8

Tom Pullen recorded that Bucheski was "doing well, although George Hendry and his SBA continued to keep a close eye on the patient."[115]

Wednesday, September 9

Happily, "Bucheski continued his convalescence with no complications, a tribute to our two man medical team's consummate professionalism." However, later that evening, the convoy was spotted and reported by U-584 at the extreme southerly end of *Gruppe Vorwärts'* screen. Thirteen U-boats were all ready to pounce.

Thursday, September 10, 1715 hours

Empire Oil, a tanker of 8000 tons sailing in ballast, was torpedoed by U-659 on her starboard side, in the way of the engine room. There was a dull thud, debris, smoke and steam rose high in the air, but there was no flash and no water thrown up.... She stopped, settling by the stern and falling off two points to starboard.... To man her armament of a 4 inch gun, a 12 pounder and an Oerlikon, *Empire Oil* carried five naval and six army (Royal Artillery) gunners.... One of the latter group, a gunlayer named Jones [not to be confused with *Ottawa's* torpedo gunner, Lloyd Irwin Jones] had been severely wounded by the explosion when a rivet was driven deep into his abdomen, causing him excruciating pain.[116]

The tanker was hit again and began to settle. Twenty-four of her crew, including the badly injured gunner, were rescued by *Ottawa* and another twenty-seven were taken off by *St. Croix.* Tom Pullen wrote:

The task of getting those twenty-four survivors up the port side and onto the iron deck went off smoothly, except for poor Jones, for whom any movement was agony. Despite the encouragement of his shipmates and the patient but determined work of our "troops," it was slow work. To the Captain [Rutherford] it must have seemed forever because, of course, we had to remain stopped and vulnerable to attack. Not once were we hectored from the bridge for the delay. I admired him for that. Finally, when able to report all clear, the water under our counter was quickly transformed into a maelstrom by our screws. To everyone's relief, we were off and running.

This was the situation on board *Ottawa* at 2100 hours of 10 September 1942: The exploding torpedo that sank Gunner Jones's ship blew a rivet through his abdominal wall like a projectile, tearing and crushing loops of small intestine inside and possibly damaging the large bowel as well. Luckily, there seemed to have been no damage done to vascular organs like the liver, stomach, or spleen. He was not bleeding profusely and therefore was not technically in shock.

Many times during this incredible week, George Hendry must have murmured a quiet prayer of thanksgiving for the experience he had gained in abdominal surgery during 1938–39 as a senior intern (resident) at St. Michael's Hospital in downtown Toronto. Bucheski's appendectomy had certainly been an invaluable dress rehearsal, but now the daunting prospect of repairing Gunner Jones's horrendous injuries was really going to put this skill to the test.

In order to grasp the difficulties that George Hendry had to overcome in carrying out the operations that he did, one must try to imagine the almost galactic differences that exist between the operative management of massive abdominal trauma in a twenty-first-century university hospital during peacetime, completely undisturbed by the weather outside, and the same surgery done in 1942 on a moving target, a poor seaman who'd had his intestine torn up by an exploding rivet and who'd been lashed to the dining table in the tiny captain's day cabin of a destroyer rolling in ten-foot mid-Atlantic seas. And all this time, the ship is scurrying around trying to hunt down any one of thirteen German submarines attacking the convoy it was escorting.

Recently, on a ferry in a calmer sea in the Bay of Fundy between Saint John and Digby, I stood against a small table and tried to imagine myself attempting some relatively simple surgical procedure. I'd had over forty years' experience as a surgeon but I had difficulty keeping my balance, let alone contemplating more demanding operative skills. At that point, my admiration for George Hendry grew by leaps and bounds.

Even in 1942, there was an obvious difference between carrying out major abdominal surgery in a large urban or university hospital and the prospect of doing the same work in a small ship in wartime. True, the big-city surgeon then had no antibiotics other than sulphathiazole, one of the very first sulphonamides, given by mouth or sprinkled into wounds or the peritoneal cavity at operation. The newly discovered penicillin would not be available for medical use by intramuscular or intravenous injection until mid-1944. Blood transfusion was a crude procedure fraught with danger, and the anaesthesia of the time was very limited and unsophisticated. The surgeon on land did, however, have a scrupulously clean working environment within his hospital, trained operating room assistants, a ready array of surgical instruments, and the basic X-ray machines of the day.

When confronted with serious intestinal injuries, today's surgeons can tap a wide array of resources. Provided that the patient is not in shock caused by excessive blood loss, the nature and extent of these wounds can be readily assessed by such diagnostic procedures as intravenous pyelography, diagnostic peritoneal lavage, ultrasound, CT scans (computerized axial tomography), MRI (magnetic resonance imaging), diagnostic laparoscopy, and biochemical determinations that accurately assess fluid and electrolyte status. Then, before, during, and after the necessary surgical procedure, these people have at hand advanced methods of intravenous fluid and drug administration, a wide range of antibiotics, safe blood replacement, state-of-the-art operating suites with the latest instruments, and sophisticated anaesthesia administration and monitoring equipment. They have skilled residents and anaesthesiologists to assist them and experienced consultants close by. Most importantly, these surgeons have the capacity to proceed immediately.

It will certainly come as no surprise that George Hendry had none of these blessings on board *Ottawa*. He had a little makeshift operating room with improvised lighting, crude ether anaesthesia, no antibiotics other than some sulphathiozole powder, a bare minimum of surgical instruments, no suction equipment (essential for this kind of operation), risky blood transfusion capability, and primitive equipment for intravenous fluid and blood administration. His only skilled help was his sick berth attendant, Alex MacMillan. No matter how inexpert, his other assistants (like Tom Pullen) were certainly willing.

For more than fifty years, Canadian surgical practice had been influenced, almost exclusively, by renowned British leaders of the discipline like Rodney Maingot, whose teaching emphasized the exercise of judgement and sturdy, unequivocal principles. Like Osler, they made elegant prose and pithy memorable aphorism their teaching method.

Experience had shown that if the necessary surgery was delayed beyond twelve hours, 70 percent of patients with these injuries would die.[117] Maingot could put this point more eloquently: "A penetrating wound in the abdomen probably means a penetrating wound of the bowel or other abdominal viscus, and demands the earliest intervention, unless a wisdom of prescience born of great experience justifies restraint."[118]

George Hendry knew this from his experience at St. Michael's Hospital before the war, but he had no choice but to wait until things settled down a bit outside. At least seven of *Gruppe Vorwärts'* thirteen U-boats were attacking the convoy under cover of darkness, and *Ottawa*, together with her sister escort warships, was fully involved in hunting down these marauders all night long, however unsuccessfully. Furthermore, Dr. Hendry and SBA MacMillan had their hands full in sick bay and elsewhere. Poor Jones was in agony despite repeated injections of morphine, and, according to a survivor's account after *Ottawa*'s sinking,[119] he had to be given a blood transfusion. Some of the other men rescued from *Empire Oil* had wounds needing treatment. Over and above that, Gunner (T) Lloyd Jones, Electrical Artificer Hobbis, and others had to help Hendry and MacMillan rig the captain's day cabin again for surgery. As Tom Pullen wrote, this operation "promised to be a messier business than the appendectomy."

Late in the morning of September 11, 1942, it was the same scenario as Pooch Bucheski's operation. There were still ten-foot seas, the patient was strapped down to the little dining table in the captain's day cabin, and Tom Pullen's "services as helper were requested as volunteers were in short supply, except, of course, for SBA MacMillan"[120] who took over the ether anaesthetic once Dr. Hendry had it started. Now the abdomen was painted with alcohol-iodine and draped with sterile towels around its perimeter.

By mid-afternoon of September 11, at the same time that Gunner Jones was undergoing his surgical ordeal, at least seven German submarines were closing in. U-584 and U-404 gained attacking positions ahead of the convoy. U-584, skillfully avoiding detection, fired two torpedoes, one of which hit the 4,884-ton SS *Hindanger. Arvida* obtained a doubtful echo and fired a ten-charge pattern that failed to find its target. *Ottawa* also made contact and fired a second pattern but her depth charges also exploded harmlessly above U-584. The convoy then made an emergency turn to port while both *Ottawa* and *Arvida* swept across the stern of the formation without making contact. At the same time, U-91, U-92, U-608, U-380, and U-211 were in the vicinity but were unable to launch successful attacks when the convoy made its evasive turns.

So that the reader can fully appreciate George Hendry's incredible accomplishment that day, it will be necessary to get into a little more technically explicit detail.[121] In cases like these, the abdomen was always opened through a long, vertical, so-called "paramedian" incision much longer than the appendectomy incision and separate from the exploding rivet's entry wound, to prevent contamination. Of course, no record of the operation survived, but it seems from Tom Pullen's colourful description[122] that these rivet injuries were found in the many loops of small intestine packed into the centre of the abdominal cavity. The first step would have been to search very gingerly for the embedded rivet and to remove it without stirring anything up. The man was not in shock and there apparently was no active bleeding. There certainly was no suction apparatus on board, so George Hendry would have had to rely on gauze pads or "sponges" to mop up any blood or intestinal fluid upon opening the peritoneum that lines the abdominal cavity.

Now, the small intestine is rather like a very soft fifteen-foot garden hose, one to two inches in diameter, suspended or slung from a fan-like membrane called a mesentery, which is compressed in folds like an accordion and literally packed into the abdominal cavity. A projectile like this rivet could (and did) damage by crushing and tearing the bowel wall, its supporting mesentery, and the blood vessels within that supply the intestine. If the mesentery was torn, a segment of small intestine would lose its blood supply and die.

The bowel itself might be lacerated, spilling out intestinal fluid. Each tear had to be found and repaired. Any segment of bowel that looked purple, as though it had lost its blood supply, would have to be resected (cut out) and the two severed ends very carefully sutured together. Because it does not lie centrally like the small intestine, injury to the large bowel (caecum and colon) is much less likely, but when it does, leakage of E. Coliladen faeces can lead to lethal peritonitis.

Here is Tom Pullen's account of the operation as performed by George Hendry, replete with its colourful nautical metaphor:

146

In the event, it was a surgical tour de force as Doc hauled out segment after segment of intestine, making the necessary repairs then re-stowing the lot in an exhausting performance lasting more than four hours. It was rather like overhauling a boat's falls. Cut and stitch. Cut and stitch. It was grisly and it did not seem possible that a stomach could accommodate so much running rigging. I emerged from what was an ordeal for all concerned with increased respect for George Hendry. What we would have done without him is difficult to imagine. Once again, his outstanding efforts were reported to the Captain.[123]

At the end of the procedure, George sprinkled in whatever sulphathiozole powder he had into the peritoneal cavity without much hope that it would do any good. He would have closed the long incision with heavier so-called retention sutures (if indeed he had any on hand) to prevent the weakened abdomen from bursting post-operatively.

Hendry undoubtedly knew that, despite all his efforts, peritonitis would be inevitable and poor Jones had little chance of survival, but of course this likelihood didn't deter him. Because of the nature of the injury, the conditions for the surgery, the time interval between the injury and the surgery, and the fact that antibiotics were non-existent at that point in the war, it is not at all surprising that the cause of this man's death was generalized peritonitis. In 1943, on land in Sicily, with far better staffed and equipped Field Surgical Units, the mortality rate for patients with blunt and penetrating abdominal trauma was 54 percent.[124]

Saturday, September 12

"During the day," T.C. Pullen wrote, "the escort successfully held the pack at bay and in the process one of our ships damaged U-659. Among other duties, it was my business to keep the bridge informed as to the state of our patients. For the first time, I sensed that with the Captain, as with the Doctor, exhaustion was a matter for concern."[125]

Now in the throes of unavoidable peritonitis, Jones was sinking. Hendry and MacMillan fought a losing fight with whatever intravenous glucose-saline they had left, and with whatever improvised nasogastric suction to prevent any post-operative ileus (loss of peristalsis or forward intestinal motion) they could, and, of course, morphine for his pain. They kept at this all day and all night.

Sunday, September 13, 1100 hours

Not unexpectedly, according to a disappointed and very weary George Hendry, our patient died during the forenoon as a consequence of peritonitis. At sunset, all officers and hands who could be spared, including his *Empire Oil* shipmates, gathered on the quarterdeck. There, to the best of my ability, I conducted a solemn burial service from the Book of Common Prayer and Gunner Jones was committed to the deep. What it may have lacked in ceremonial was more than made good by our collective sincerity. Within a few hours, most of those attending — bareheaded and bowed — and all but one of his shipmates, would themselves be committed to the deep, in unimaginably violent circumstances.[126]

All in all, it had been a superb but exhausting performance. Typical of the man, George Hendry just got on with the job, right to the end.

"She Was a Fine Ship, Number One"

At 2000 local time (Zulu[127] minus one hour) on September 13, 1942, HMCS *Ottawa* was "slipping along at 10 knots in station 5000 yards ahead of the starboard wing of the convoy." Sub-Lieutenant Yogi Jenson, the ship's gunnery and RDF (radar) officer, wrote that he

> went on watch[128] at 8.00 p.m. [2000] with Mr. Lloyd Jones, our Torpedo Gunner and a very fine officer.[129] It was a clear, dark evening, becoming overcast. The sea was fairly calm, but a westerly breeze was getting up. Most of the time we could just discern the ships in the convoy, but as we patrolled back and forth on our station, we could check that all was well. *St. Croix* and *Ottawa* were getting low on fuel, but we were supposed to be relieved [soon] by two destroyers out of St. John's, HMS *Witch* and HMCS *Annapolis*.[130]

Since morning, one more ship, the Panamanian *Stonestreet*, had been torpedoed and sunk by U-594 with the loss of thirteen men. This was the seventh ship to be lost so far, plus four damaged but still able to make way.

At 1505, a Catalina flying boat piloted by Flying-Officer R.M. MacLennan of RCAF 116 Squadron out of Botwood, Newfoundland, arrived overhead and forced three of the attackers to submerge: U-96, U-411, and U-380. This aircraft was operating at its maximum range from base, 550 miles; the convoy was indeed all but out of the Black Pit.

In mid-morning, a disappointed and extremely tired George Hendry reported the almost inevitable death of *Empire Oil's* DEMS Gunner Jones from post-operative peritonitis complicating his horrendous intestinal injuries. One of *Ottawa's* survivors, Lieutenant Dunn Lantier, said later that George Hendry had worked "like a Trojan on two cases he would have been lucky to save if he had had a city hospital's facilities at his disposal."[131]

Coming off watch at 1600, Jenson and Lloyd Jones were having a cup of tea in the wardroom when the First Lieutenant Tom Pullen broke the news that Gunner Jones would be buried at sea that afternoon.

"At about 1645," Jenson wrote, "all hands not on watch were piped to fall in on the Quarterdeck. The body in its canvas shroud was laid out on a six-foot wooden plank, covered with a large White Ensign. The burial service was read by the First Lieutenant, the honour guard then fired three volleys, six men hoisted the plank and the body slid from beneath the ensign into the sea. It was a quiet wardroom at supper that evening."[132]

By 2000, back on watch on the bridge, Jenson heard the ASDIC pinging away "as it always did at sea, searching steadily either side of our bow," but because any submarines in the immediate vicinity of the ship would be stealing in on the surface under cover of darkness, there were no echoes. *Ottawa's* unreliable Type 286M radar "swept complete circles around the ship, but it could not be depended on even to show the convoy much less any lurking submarines."[133]

In mid-1942, only Royal Navy ships had the vastly superior Type 271 centimetric radar sets, and thus HMS *Celandine* was the only ship in C-4 escort group to be so equipped. It came as a stroke of very bad luck that her 271 set was unserviceable late on Sunday evening, September 13, 1942.

Jenson found this duty completely routine: "The lookouts, on either side of the bridge, constantly searching through their binoculars, saw nothing but the blackness of night. Jones and I drank cocoa and gave helm orders, zig-zagging on our random patrol. It was a typical night watch."[134]

AB Roe Skillen and his shipmates were very tired:

When day broke on September 13, 1942, the *Ottawa* had been in action since 1200 hours on the 10th. The wolf-pack had managed to infiltrate the escort and had sunk 6 or 7 ships of the convoy. To the crew of the *Ottawa*, it was either watch stations or action stations and fatigue was starting to set in. We had left our station more than once to respond to an ASDIC alert or to check something that loomed ahead of the convoy. Rest was out of the question, but as the day passed, our spirits were buoyed by the "buzz" that we were to be relieved before midnight. I was to go on watch at 2400 hours. Some of the watch crawled into their "micks" [hammocks] while some of us tried to pass the time playing cards. About 2300 hours, I decided to try and catch a few winks, so two or three of us crashed on the deck next to the hammock rack.[135]

At 2252, the radar operator reported two strong contacts at Green 30° (or about 30° on the starboard bow), one at eight thousand and one at six thousand yards. With the ship's sadly deficient radar set, Yogi Jenson was frustrated: "It could well have been Red 150°, the reciprocal bearing!" The range of the suspicious contact continued to close. As a precaution, just in case it actually was a submarine creeping in, a five-charge pattern of depth charges, set to explode at fifty feet, was readied and the ship's speed increased to twelve knots and a little later to fifteen knots. At this time, the ASDIC operator reported HE (hydrophone effect[136]), but this was assumed to be from the screws of the approaching *Witch*. He was ordered to disregard this. Tom Pullen wrote:

> There was no reply, but it was correctly assumed the contacts were *Witch* and *Annapolis*, the two destroyers coming to relieve oil-depleted *Ottawa* and *St. Croix*. The signalman made <AA> ("What ship?") on Green 30° and a tiny flash back said "Witch." By then the range was down to five cables [one thousand yards] and in view of *Witch*'s proximity, Jenson suggested to the Captain [who had just been called to the bridge] that "perhaps we should alter

away." The Captain agreed with the alteration, so I said "Port 15" to the quartermaster, who repeated the order and the ship started to turn to port, about 20 degrees.[137]

The radar operator reported a faint echo on the port bow, but he wasn't very sure about it. Because of the acknowledged weakness of the radar, he probably assumed that this was a fallacious reciprocal radar contact of the rapidly oncoming *Witch*, when in fact it may have been a contact accurately identifying an approaching submarine.

In his memoirs written forty-eight years later, Tom Pullen explained:

> It was the German practice to attack en masse on the surface under cover of dark, charging at the convoy from ahead and passing down between the columns, firing torpedoes as they went. Once in the convoy's wake, they [would] make good their escape submerging only if threatened. During daylight, when safely below the horizon, they would surface and overtake the convoy to position themselves for a repeat performance. With air support, of course, it was possible during daylight to frustrate such tactics. Accordingly, the likeliest place to encounter U-boats after dark was five or ten miles in the grain[138] of a convoy, lying in wait to renew the nightly fireworks. This was the danger zone into which *Ottawa* was heading and where it is possible that she became fatally distracted by the approaching destroyers. Had we been fitted with radar Type 271 (as we should have been but were not because there was not time or some such excuse), the lurking enemy would most likely have been detected and the tables turned. It is also possible during those final minutes on our bridge, [our] lookouts were concentrating on the radar targets. It is equally possible that because the dark was so dark, nothing could have been seen of a skulking submarine trimmed down and probably end-on, no matter how vigilant our lookouts.[139]

So it was that three minutes after 2300, concealed by darkness a mile or so to port, Oberleutnant zur See Heinz Walkerling, the commanding officer of U-91, was surprised to find himself in the near vicinity of three escorts and ideally placed to attack undetected: "I sight several silhouettes and must be positioned directly ahead of the convoy. I discern a twin-funnelled destroyer at slow speed far ahead of the convoy on inclination 70."[140]

Earlier that evening, Tom Pullen found that he could almost wax lyrical: "All was tranquil. The sea lay calm beneath a starry sky and the familiar swishing sounds of our bow wave fell gently away from the shoulders of the ship.... Apart from the ticking of the gyro [compass] repeat and the tireless pinging of the ASDIC, all seemed peaceful. I went aft to rest in preparation for my morning watch."

Resting in his bunk, Pullen "sensed our two increases in speed.... When the revolutions went from twelve to fifteen knots, my curiosity was fully aroused (a sudden increase could mean a submarine contact, action stations and a general hubbub)." As he was making a sandwich for Lieutenant Pullen down the corridor in *Ottawa's* wardroom pantry, Leading Steward Michael Barriault also felt the ship surge ahead. Quickly, Tom Pullen slid on his sea boots, and "went up … onto the quarterdeck to investigate. All was serene: dark, no moon, no breeze, an oily-looking sea, smooth with a barely perceptible swell. I spotted a signal lamp winking off in the distance and read the word *Witch*.... I heard in the background: 'Port 15.' The ship began to swing in that direction heeling ever so slightly to starboard as she went."[141]

As entered in U-91's torpedo shot report, or *Schussmeldung*,[142] a salvo of two torpedoes was fired at 2303 from Tubes I and III at a speed of eleven knots, a depth of two meters, a spread angle of four degrees, a range of one thousand metres, and a running time of forty-five seconds. It was all very precise and the target was midships (*mitte*) of *Ottawa's* port side.

"Two explosions after 1 minute 50 seconds." Two torpedoes had indeed been fired but only one, and not two, as Walkerling thought, had hit the target. "Black and white explosive cloud and bright red flames. The destroyer stopped burning heavily and fires a shell which splits into 5 green stars."[143]

At 2305, there was a huge explosion. Yogi Jenson, standing watch on the bridge, saw an amazing geranium-coloured flash forward, followed by a great pillar of water which went straight up. All of us then took shelter under the overhang at the front of the bridge, while the water and all sorts of solid objects tumbled down from the sky. When the downpour stopped, I went back to the compass [platform] and we stopped engines. The ship lay still in the water, rocking gently. The fo'c'sle, with anchors and chains, together with "A" gun[144] had vanished. The forward canopy, with "B" gun, drooped down toward the water. These features were visible because the interior lights were all on and shining out over the ocean. We obviously were a particularly lovely target, so the engines were ordered slow astern. A number of British destroyers had suffered similar damage and some had been able to make port by going astern much of the way.[145]

Tom Pullen hesitated:

Following that night-shattering eruption, nothing broke the silence, no shouts, no alarm bells. Even the sound of the sea rippling against the ship's side … as the engines stopped…. Now training asserted itself and, tumbling below to my cabin, I grabbed my flashlight, knife, morphine, pistol, flask and lifebelt…. As fast as my legs could carry me, I legged it for the bridge. The scene greeting me on reaching the compass platform was memorable. Forward of "B" gun, there was nothing but water. The bow, including "A" gun and all, had vanished and the blast screen between "A" and "B" guns was folded back on itself…. Hesitating just long enough to report to the Captain, I headed below to assess the situation…. Getting to the scene of damage would have been impossible without my flashlight. The narrow passage leading to the messdecks [seamen's quarters in the fo'c'sle or forward section of the ship] was jammed with survivors in shock stumbling out on to the upper deck…. Clattering down the ladder into the stokers' mess, or what remained of it … all was chaos and carnage. Fortunately, the torpedo just missed the forward 4.7 inch magazine or half the ship or more, not just the bow, would have gone "galley west" ("Navy" for "would have been obliterated"). The adjacent messdeck forward, what had been the fore-lower messdeck for Signalmen and Telegraphists, had disappeared completely, being replaced by a view of the Atlantic. Nothing remained. The space that had been the stokers' living quarters had been transformed into a waist-high jumble of damaged lockers, mess tables, hammocks, clothing; all framed by torn and twisted steel. Underneath the wreckage could be heard groans from a few victims who had survived the blast and were in great distress. Above me were the bloody remains of lifeless men smashed upwards from their hammocks and impaled on overhead fittings by the tremendous force of the explosion. In the light of my torch, the battered face, or what remained of it, of one familiar stoker was barely recognizable. The Doctor [George Hendry] and the Chief Engineer [D.L. McGillivray] appeared and together we tried to assess this scene of death and devastation.[146]

At 2305, when the first torpedo struck, Steve Logos, who was scheduled to stand middle watch (midnight to 0400), was in his hammock "getting some much needed rest":

I slept in at least my shirt, pants and socks with my seaboots stowed underneath my hammock. The jolt of the torpedo knocked me right up against the bulkhead and eventually I would need a couple of stitches in my head. I picked up my duffel coat as I ran for the quarterdeck. My position at "Action Stations" was to be in charge of the two rows of depth charges at the very stern of the ship. I was the one who set the depth of the explosion and dropped them off the ship as per instructions.... Gunner [Lloyd] Jones then arrived and we took it upon ourselves to remove the primers and throw them overboard to make sure the depth charges did not go off [when the ship sank].... Actually the primers were in safe position, but we took no chances. So, about 75 depth charges on the quarterdeck were rendered safe. [147]

This prompt action saved many lives, for, had it not been taken, the underwater explosion of armed depth charges as the ship sank would have caused fatal blast immersion injuries to men in the water.

AB Sid Dobing "was standing at the after end of the bridge, where my duties were to act as a communicator between the bridge and the quarterdeck where the depth charge crews were stationed." When the first torpedo struck,

I was knocked off my feet as a huge wave of water swamped the bridge. I picked myself up and found a large piece of metal, probably a part of the bows, lying at my feet. The phone from the quarterdeck rang within minutes and it was Lloyd Jones, the Gunner (T), in a calm voice, instructing me to report to the Captain that all depth charges had been rendered safe. Some ships had been sunk when this hadn't been done, resulting in death to survivors when they exploded. Lloyd's calm and reassuring voice gave me a lot of self-confidence and many years later I was able to tell him how much that had meant to me at the time.[148]

AB Alvin Underhill survived the sinking precisely because Pooch Bucheski had had to be operated upon for acute appendicitis: "Bucheski would have been on 'B' gun as captain if he had not been taken ill. I would have been in my hammock port side, which is where the first torpedo hit. However, the Gunner's Mate, PO Grivel, informed me at 1600 that I would assume that position [gun captain] from 2000 to midnight and the first torpedo hit at approximately 2300, taking off the bow section of the ship just ahead of 'B' gun!"[149]

In the upper after messdeck, Yogi Jenson found

> a group of about twenty men … clustered by a hammock netting. A number of them were terribly wounded, many with grossly twisted limbs; it was like a scene from hell.
>
> I then started aft, along the upper deck, encountering first the Surgeon [George Hendry], then the First Lieutenant [Tom Pullen] … and finally Sub-Lieutenant [Donald] Wilson, recently joined, who had just taken over the Confidential Books from me, that is the codes and ciphers, intelligence and other secret documents. He understood that it was his duty to put all of these in weighted bags and drop them overboard. I tried to convince him not to go below again as I feared another "fish" (torpedo). He would not be convinced and, despite my pleading, went below decks to do as he intended.[150]

Just as Yogi feared, Wilson didn't make it out of the sinking ship.

Over on the other side of the convoy, five thousand yards ahead of the port column, the weary captain of *St. Croix*, Lieutenant Commander Andrew Hedley Dobson ("Hedley" to his family; "Dobbie" to his friends), went to his sea cabin and, for the first time since leaving Lough Foyle, took off his seaboots before lying down. Just as his head hit the pillow, the voice pipe recalled him urgently to the bridge. A message from *Witch* handed to him there read: "Believe *Ottawa* torpedoed." At that moment, "two white rockets" exploded in the distance over by *Ottawa*. Dobson gave his orders quietly: "Action Stations. Ring on full ahead both. Starboard 10 to 280." *St. Croix* sheered off at speed to come to the aid of her sister ship on the other side of the convoy.[151, 152] She swept up to *Ottawa's* starboard side, slowed, pulled abeam of where the destroyer's bow should have been, and stopped. It was precisely 2319.

The entry from the ROP (Report of Proceedings) of HMS *Witch* for 0003Z (2303 local time), September 14, 1942:

With *Witch* in position approximately 270 degrees, 10,000 yards from leading ship of starboard wing column, *Ottawa* was silhouetted by a large explosion, which appeared to take place in the vicinity of the port side of her after funnel. *Witch*, assuming *Ottawa* to be torpedoed, fired two white rockets, informed *St. Croix* (CTU 24.1.14) by R/T that *Ottawa* was believed to be torpedoed. Course was immediately altered and a sweep carried out across the head of the convoy to the port bow, back to the vicinity of *Ottawa*, and down the starboard side of convoy.[153]

Heinz Walkerling's KTB entry (KTB is short for *Kriegstagebuch*: war diary) immediately after the first torpedo struck reads: "Starshells are ... fired from other vessels. I assume that this is an emergency signal as a second destroyer proceeds to the position from which it was fired. I turn a full circle using maximum helm and commence a new approach towards the second destroyer which is now lying stopped. Fired single shot [at 2318] from Tube II with firing angle zero degrees. Running time one minute, 45 seconds."[154]

The target was again midships, but this time it was the starboard side of the ship. At 2320, the U-91's second torpedo passed just underneath *St. Croix*'s counter, and its massive explosion tore a huge gap in *Ottawa*'s starboard side just abaft no. 2 boiler, cutting the mortally wounded destroyer in two. In the confusion of the moment, Walkerling thought he had hit *St. Croix* instead and thus claimed two destroyers sunk in his report.[155]

It has been suggested that *Witch*, and not *St. Croix*, was the second destroyer that Walkerling thought he had torpedoed. The ROPs from both Dobson[156] and Woods[157] make it quite clear that *St. Croix* was the target.

Now acutely aware of being the next available target, *St. Croix* pulled ahead quickly and turned back down *Ottawa*'s port side. Dobson ordered *Celandine* and *Arvida* to pick up survivors and then *St. Croix* left the area to conduct sweeps in an attempt to track down *Ottawa*'s killer.[158, 159]

Jenson, back on the bridge, "found the Captain and the First Lieutenant engaged in firing a rocket, a signal that we had been torpedoed. At that very moment, a second torpedo hit us, this time in the region of

No. 2 Boiler Room [behind the bridge and underneath the forward funnel]. A huge flash and then water deluging down on us. It was immediately apparent that the ship was doomed. She settled in the water and the Captain called out to abandon ship."[160]

Tom Pullen recalled:

> Everything happened so quickly. I left my cabin to investigate the second speed increase at 2300. At 2305, came the first torpedo, followed at 2320 by the second. The latter exploded in Number Two Boiler Room, located between the two funnels, starboard side, wreaking havoc and breaking her back.... The forward part where we were started to submerge and commenced listing to starboard. From the grinding, tearing sounds all about, the ship was breaking up. There was nothing to be done but clear out in what few seconds remained. I followed Chief and Doc up the ladder to the Seamen's Mess. In the renewed confusion, the ship heeling amid the roar of escaping steam, it was a monumental struggle getting up the inside ladder to the bridge, parting on the way from George Hendry on the flagdeck. I never saw him again.[161]

Radar Operator AB Terry Terrabassi was asleep in his hammock on the lower seamen's messdeck when the first torpedo struck and blew the bow off the ship. He heard no alarm and "action stations" was not piped. The messdeck was a gruesome sight: it was torn apart and there were mangled, dismembered bodies everywhere. Miraculously, Terrabassi was unhurt, but one of his shipmates who had been playing cards a few feet away had been cut in two by the explosion.

Suddenly, Terry remembered that, in the imminent event of a ship's sinking, Admiralty Standing Orders required that the radar equipment be thrown overboard to prevent its falling into enemy hands. So he rushed to the radar shack abaft the bridge, clambering over bodies — dead and alive — as fast as he could. On the bridge, an officer (Terrabassi can't recall who) denied his request to ditch the radar set, insisting that the wounded ship might well survive by going astern. It was at this point that the second torpedo exploded amidships, breaking the ship's back, and she began to sink quickly.

Terry recalls this was the only time that he was really scared — so much so that he was trembling uncontrollably. What remained of *Ottawa's* fo'c'sle rolled over, and Terry walked down its side and jumped into the sea. As he was doing this, he shouted to no one in particular, "Wait for me!"

By the time Tom Pullen got back to the bridge, the ship's back was broken and she was already beginning to roll over on her beam ends. The order to abandon ship was passed. Pullen described the preparations for this final procedure:

> Altogether, we carried nine Carley floats for a ship's company of 180 officers and men, or 20 to a float. This meant overcrowding but it had to be assumed that in the unhappy eventuality, this would be offset by casualties. There were the two 27 foot whalers and the 25 foot motorboat but destroyers are so slightly built and torpedoes wreak such damage, there is rarely time to get undamaged boats (like these) away in time.... Despite the loss of seventy or so men already, there was still over-crowding, so much so that some overburdened floats capsized, throwing their exhausted occupants into the water and adding to the death toll.
>
> During those final moments, there were some grim dramas being played out. The pitiable entreaties emanating from the voice pipe to the bridge from the two young hands trapped in the ASDIC hut far below became unbearable to those of us on the bridge, who were totally helpless to do anything for them. What could, what should, one do other than offer words of encouragement that help was coming, when such was manifestly out of the question? What happened at the end is hard to contemplate for the imprisoned pair, as that pitch black, watertight, soundproofed box rolled first 90 degrees to starboard and then 90 degrees on to

its back before sliding into the depths and oblivion. It is an ineradicable memory.

Then there was Bucheski [the appendectomy patient], on whose behalf, *our gallant doctor,* with SBA MacMillan and Pooch's friends, dedicated themselves to the task of saving him. Tragically, they opted for the starboard whaler which was directly in the line of fire when the second torpedo arrived, annihilating everyone and everything in the vicinity. For those struggling to lower the boat, death must have been instantaneous. Mr. [Lloyd] Jones, our redoubtable Gunner (T), slightly removed from that scene was blown overboard but unhurt, and somehow managed to climb back on board by a scrambling net.[162]

Others were just as sure as Tom Pullen had been that the surgeon, his assistant, his patient, and his patient's friends were gone in a flash. Sid Dobing had witnessed this selfless act from the bridge.

And Al Underhill remembers that "Norm Soles [his friend and shipmate] and I had observed that quite a number of people had gathered at the … whaler, and we assumed and later confirmed that Dr. Hendry and members of the crew were assisting to place AB Bucheski in the … whaler in case the ship went down. It was at this time that the second torpedo struck in this area and we assumed that the Doctor and the crew assisting him were all killed."[163]

After being rescued, Lieutenant Dunn Lantier remembered "Dr. Hendry and two others … going to put him [Bucheski] in one of the whalers but both were smashed [by the second torpedo explosion], and we never saw him again. As for the Doctor, I never saw him either."[164]

But Gunner (T) Lloyd Jones did. "He was on my float.[165] I remember he was full of good spirits, trying to cheer the rest of us. But after a while we drifted out of the oil-covered area and a big sea came up. The raft capsized three or four times, and we all had to scramble in the dark to get back to it. Lieutenant Hendry was able to get back and hang on the first three times, but the next time we got overturned, he just didn't get back."[166]

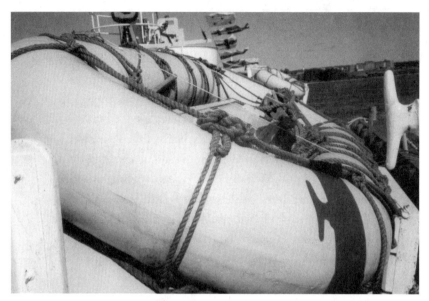

Typical Carley float on HMCS Sackville. *Note the rope lanyards bound closely to the sides of the float. Exhausted men found it extremely difficult, if not impossible, to hold onto them in rough seas. (Courtesy of Dr. James Goodwin.)*

After jumping in from the sinking *Ottawa*, Terry Terrabassi swam to the nearest Carley float. It was a pitch black night and the sea was getting up. There were twenty-two cold, bone-tired men clinging to this particular float, and Dr. George Hendry was one of them. Terry knew that Hendry was utterly exhausted after operating on two sailors and caring for them continuously over the past four days. Each time the float flipped over in the rough sea, Terry saw that the doctor had great difficulty grasping the lanyard again. Finally, the fourth time the float capsized, George Hendry couldn't hold on and he was swept away in the dark.

It was just after 2300, when Roe Skillen was

> lying there on the deck wondering when our relief [HMS *Witch* and HMCS *Annapolis*] would arrive…. I felt a thump as if something had heaved below me. Then "Action Stations" rang out. I headed out past the break of the fo'c'sle and up the ladder on the upper deck to the .50 calibre machine guns. There were three of us up there. An eerie silence fell over the ship. We were dead in the water,

knew we had been hit but did not know how badly. After some minutes had passed, the order was given to leave our position and help with the wounded. I was last in line and as I stepped on the first rung, a terrible explosion broke the silence.

The next thing I knew I was lying on the starboard side, aft of the rear stack, and up against the guard rail. I don't know how long I had been "out", but I felt I might be the only one left aboard. My right leg was jammed against a stanchion and I tried to free myself, but to no avail. That was when I thought I would die. I said a prayer asking God to forgive me. I thought of my family and my fiancée who would be left to mourn but something urged me to try again. My leg did come loose and I slipped over the side into a dark and foreboding Atlantic. I gazed over to where our ship was slowly sinking and I realized that I had to get away as fast as I could. Because I had always been told about the chance of suction taking you down as the ship went down.[167]

After attending the burial service for poor Jones (the DEMS gunlayer from *Empire Oil*), Stoker George Johnson "returned to the Stokers' mess, changed into my steaming gear and went on watch [at 2000] in the engine room. Then about 2300, the first torpedo struck us forward in the area of the communications [signalmen's and telegraphists'] mess." The first torpedo had blown off *Ottawa's* bow ahead of "B" gun. The stokers' mess was immediately below "B" gun, and it's not surprising that its ceiling was badly damaged by the blast. A hurried order was given to install bracing timbers there and Johnson "was sent forward to report on how the shoring ... was progressing. I reached the break of the fo'c'sle port side when the second torpedo struck # 2 Boiler Room. It then became 'abandon ship'. My Carley float was on the quarterdeck, but it was already in the water. I came back to where the torpedo tubes were located and three of us tried to free another float there, but no success." The ship had been cut in two, and as its stern section was lying on its starboard side, "three of us walked down her port side and into the water."[168]

It was an immense piece of luck that AB Edward Fox was off duty that night and was asleep in his hammock in the seamen's messdeck. He was an ASDIC operator and was spared the awful fate of two of his mates who were trapped and drowned in the ASDIC cabinet deep in the belly of the ship when its door was jammed shut by the explosion of the first torpedo. It was their frantic screams that Yogi Jenson and Tom Pullen heard coming up the bridge voice pipe.

As it was, Fox was blown against the messdeck bulkhead by that first torpedo blast, deeply lacerating his side and cracking several ribs. Because of an unpopular standing order, ratings were to wear their awkward, cumbersome lifebelts at all times, even when off duty. In his battered and dazed state, Edward probably owed his life to this regulation, for he's still not sure how he got into the sea that night.

"To those of us on the bridge," Tom Pullen wrote, "it was obvious that the end was coming, and rapidly. Only a few seconds remained to put a few hurried puffs into what passed for lifejackets in those days."[169] Tom Pullen had one; Larry Rutherford didn't. In an act of magnificent selflessness, he'd given his to a rating without one.

> Together the Captain and I scrambled out of the bridge, into the port sponson, and from there onto the ship's side.... We picked our way carefully, pausing when we reached the bilge keel. As we stood side by side, hesitating, his quiet last words to me were: "*She was a fine ship, Number One.*" He jumped and I followed. When I plunged, clutching my flashlight and burdened by that heavy pistol, my water-filled seaboots dragged me straight down. Struggling to get rid of them took some seconds, all the while being pulled deeper. Finally kicking them clear, I surfaced, but by then Larry Rutherford was nowhere to be seen. It was dark, the sea blanketed with oil making it impossible to identify individuals. I never encountered him again. After four days and nights of unremitting stress, he was really beyond coping with the physical demands involved in continuing the struggle. Also, he was wearing a lammy coat, heavier and more

water-absorbent than duffel, a deadly encumbrance had he not shucked it.[170]

Under these circumstances, then, a lifebelt probably wouldn't have saved Rutherford.

Tom Pullen was fully aware that "it was urgent to distance oneself from the wreck, but progress through a thick layer of Bunker C [fuel oil] was difficult. For a ship critically low in fuel, there seemed to be a great deal of it about. I managed about thirty yards or so before turning around to witness the sad finale. By then, the forward section was almost vertical, stem (or where the stem used to be) skyward. It hung motionless for a moment or two and then, without a sound, slid straight down and was gone."

Tom remembered,

> ... earlier, all hatches abaft the after bulkhead in the Engine Room had been shut tight and, for a moment, it seemed that the stern section might break free and remain afloat. It appeared buoyant. However, this was not to be. The stern tilted higher and higher. As it, too, approached the vertical, there came a mighty clatter, clouds of dust, and the entire after superstructure, "X" gun included as well as 70 depth charges, broke loose and plummeted into the sea. What remained of the hull dripping propellers and all, soon followed, leaving nothing in its wake but a bewildered collection of oil-covered swimmers and crowded Carley floats. By my waterproof watch, it was 2330.[171]

Norm Wilson, on the 2000 to 2400 watch, was closed up at the "B" gun (turret).

> At approximately 22:30, there was a contact on the radar and ... we went to check it as we were to be meeting our relief escort ... the RN destroyer HMS *Witch*. The two destroyers were ... signaling back and forth with small lights to verify who they were. As we were closing on *Witch*, the order was given for a turn to port.

In the middle of the turn, it appears that we came between *Witch* and an oncoming torpedo which had been homed in on the blue light of the *Witch*.

This torpedo hit us just aft of the bow on the port side and lifted the fo'c'sle deck up like a sardine can. I distinctly remember the power of the explosion and the water coming down on us. ... I remember hollering "Christ, we've been fished!" We went for the Carley float on the port side at our deck level and cleared it ready ... the order was given not to abandon ship as we were not sinking. In the confusion, somebody threw a life ring in the water with a calcium flare attached off the starboard side ... and when it lit, we were perfectly silhouetted making a perfect target. The second torpedo came into the [starboard] midships about 23:11, ten minutes after the first. [Wilson is in error about this.] That really rocked the ship and everything was dead quiet for a few moments except for the hissing of the steam from the boilers. The word was given to abandon ship and we pushed off. It was not long before the boat was crowded.... We kept the inside for any who were injured and we all hung on to the ropes on the outside. It was spectacle to see the ship break in half and (what remained of) the bow and the stern lift up.... She slipped under like two rods sliding in the water.[172]

"As predicted by the Captain, a second torpedo struck almost amidships and that was the end." The order to abandon ship was given, and Sid Dobing made his way

from the bridge to the after and starboard side, which was my "abandon ship" station. An effort to lodge the Carley float was already underway, but it became caught up under the guardrails and could not be freed. We gave up and jumped over the side into the cold, oil covered Atlantic. Our lifebelts were the inflated type, I had inflated mine right after the first torpedo struck and as a non-swimmer it was a lifesaver. I swam to a Carley float and held on to the side and watched as the ship made her final plunge. I remember hearing the ship's siren still sounding and the noise of the after 4.7 inch gun tearing loose from the deck.

Lt. Pullen called for three cheers for the old ship as she disappeared beneath the waves.[173]

Immediately after the second torpedo struck at 2320, Yogi Jenson realized that the ship was sinking.

I left the bridge and went to the port side of the fo'c'sle. Leading Seaman Hard was standing there. I remarked "Well, Leading Seaman Hard, I'm going." "So am I," said Hard and off he went. I jumped in and noticed a Dan buoy, a wooden spar with a watertight drum in the center, floating off the port bow. A man was clinging to it, a Jewish man from Montreal, I think, who may have lost a foot. After a few minutes, he dropped off and I was alone. My lifebelt was a Mae West,[174] a simple rubber tube which I inflated around my chest. The water was about 59° F as we were a few miles from the western edge of the Gulfstream. I kicked off my seaboots and with my spar I floated fairly comfortably.

The ship started to go down before my eyes. I could only see the stern part, tipping out of the water as the forward part sank lower and lower. Soon, the rudder and propellers were right out of the water. Next, "X" gun [4.7"] slipped out of its mounting and plunged downwards. Then the stern vanished beneath the waves. It was like a dream. Would all of us be sucked down as our ship sank? No, there was no such effect. Would our depth charges explode at the set depth, crushing our chests and killing us? Thank God and Mr. Jones, nothing happened.[175]

167

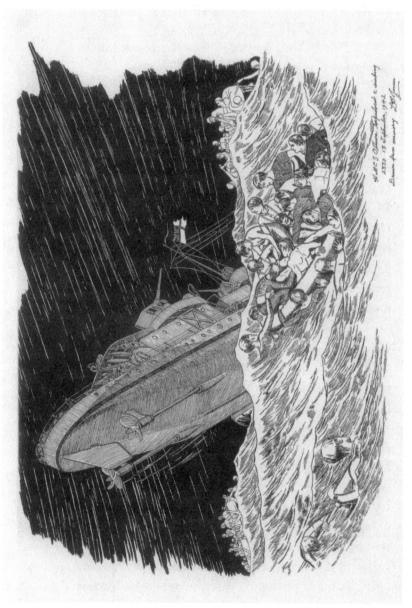

HMCS Ottawa torpedoed and sinking at 2330 on September 13, 1942. Drawn from memory by L.B. Jenson.

When it sank at 2330, September 13, 1942, the ship's position was 47° 55″ north (latitude), 43° 27″ west (longitude), roughly four hundred miles east-northeast of St. John's, Newfoundland.

> Oil started spreading out from where the ship had been; it was all over my face, my head and hands, the smell filled the air and the taste was in my mouth. Gradually, it lessened and the waves were now fresh and clean. Three or four Carley Floats bobbed around hundreds of yards away. They were crowded with men, some of whom were sitting inside the floats. But the floats kept turning over and each time there would be fewer men on the float when it righted. I decided my Dan Buoy was better than a float.
>
> I started to pray that my life would be spared, but I reasoned that would never do. I then prayed that I be given the strength to cope with my fate, whatever it might be, and recited the Lord's Prayer. In the distance, I could hear and feel depth charges exploding. The chances were that someone had a contact. [as reported in *Celandine's* ROP at 0240, "HMCS *St. Croix* was heard to be dropping depth charges in the vicinity"] But suppose the "contact" was under us! Should he attack it? I thought: "Yes, it would more important to kill the U-boat, which would only take more lives", and steeled myself to being blown up. Mercifully, the explosions became more distant and then ceased altogether.[176]

As they were sure the ship was sinking, Al Underhill and Norm Soles "slipped a cable float from the bridge area approximately 30 feet above water and then jumped in to catch hold of it. As we were on the windward side, we had to kick it astern to get clear of the ship, which would suck you in if you were too close. In a few minutes, we had 23 men hanging on to the cable float, with Roe Skillen in the center because of his badly injured leg, which was later removed in hospital."[177]

After the ship sank, Roe Skillen could hear the yelling and commotion ahead of him in the darkness, all the while hoping that the depth charges would not explode and do what the torpedoes had failed to do. I found a Carley Float and grasped a rope. I think there were at least 20 or more shipmates clinging to the sides, some crying out in pain while others voiced words of hope and encouragement. "Would anyone find us?" was on every mind. The sea, which so far had not been a factor, was beginning to whip up and I found it hard to stay awake. I remembered that as a youngster learning about exposure that you would think you were warm and cozy while you were slowly freezing to death, and all you wanted to do was fall asleep. Fortunately, the fact that the waves grew larger and we had time to time our actions, to let go of the rope when the float flipped over and then grab it again when it came down. This was enough to help us stay awake.

One by one, as time passed during the night, more of my shipmates slipped away, never to be seen again. The sea tossed the Carley Float around like an old inner tube. I think that there had been originally 22 of us clinging to it, but now there were only six of us left. Once we thought that a U-boat had surfaced near us and thought that we might be fired upon came into my head. To this day, I don't know if there was a U-boat or if my mind was playing tricks on me.[178]

After the ship sank, Sid Dobing and the others on his Carley float

tried to sort ourselves out and make sure that the injured were inside the float. Roe Skillen was one, he had a broken leg and it was impossible to make him comfortable. He had to have his leg amputated when he was finally admitted to hospital in St. John's. Among those clinging to or on the float were Lt. Pullen, Sub-Lt. Jenson, ERA Moe Locke, Petty Officer George Grivel, Stoker Harry Morrison (who died while I was trying to support him), Able Seaman

Archibald and Leading Seaman Cliff Riches (who were lost when our float overturned) and others whose names I can't remember. I believe we numbered about 20 until we lost some men after the float capsized due to the heavy swell.... Eventually, I think eight of us were rescued.[179]

When the ship began to break up and founder, Steve Logos remembers vividly that

in my case, it was off with the seaboots and jump into the water as close to a Carley float as possible. We can all thank our Maker for the fact we were sunk in the Gulf Stream where the temperature of the water was in the low sixties. If we had been sunk in the Labrador Current (just a little farther north) no one would have survived.

When I reached a Carley float, it was crowded. It seemed as if everyone was trying to get inside ... and I counted 21 on our float. The sea was rough and with too many men on the inside of the float, it would turn turtle. Unfortunately, a number would get trapped underneath it and ... would drown. With my experience at YMCA teaching swimming, I decided that it ... would be best to hang on to the rope on the outside of the float. Due to their lack of sleep having been on "Action Stations" for very lengthy periods, a number of men just did not have the stamina to hang on and they just quietly faded away in the dark. Out of the 21 that started on our Carley float, there were only five of us left when we were picked up five hours later by the *Arvida*. The story was the same for all the Carley floats.[180]

Tom Pullen was clinging to the Carley float with Skillen, Dobing, Underhill, Terrabassi, and Jenson:

It must have been around midnight when the convoy appeared silently out of the darkness, steaming majestically through our area and just as quietly was gone. A tanker in ballast passed so close, we could see a cavernous hole in her port side.

It was an exhausting night. I tried not to dwell on how long we could endure or our prospects for being picked up. The float we clung to provided support for a number of men, but as time passed, one by one they gave up and drifted wordlessly into the night. Luckily, the water was not cold, for we were still in the Gulfstream. Had we been forced to take to the water not many miles further west, we would have ended up in the frigid Labrador current, where survival time is measured in minutes, not hours. As that middle watch [0001 to 0400] dragged on, the wind strengthened, the waves grew higher, jerking me violently between Dan Buoy and the rough canvas of that unyielding float.[181]

Norm Wilson remembers, "When one is down in the water, those freighters are sure big when they pass by and you are looking up at them."[182]

As each hour passed on this bleak, desperate night, Terry Terrabassi saw that the number clinging to the float was steadily diminishing. Men were either too spent to hold on when the float repeatedly flipped over or they would quietly let go and just drift away. After a while, it began to rain gently and Terry remembers thinking, "God is so sorry about what happened out here and these rain drops are tears from Heaven." He will never forget having that thought.

They were in the upper reaches of the temperate Gulf Stream, and swarms of fist-sized jellyfish (to Terry they looked like poached eggs) bit anyone with skin exposed. Norm Wilson remembers that Terrabassi was bare-legged and severely stung by jellyfish, and when he was rescued he was given several injections of morphine for the excruciating pain.[183] But the doctor on *Celandine* and the staff at the RCN Hospital in St. John's could not accept the fact that Terrabassi was covered with jellyfish bites. These lesions had to be "calcium flare burns" or "a wire injury."

To Yogi Jenson's astonishment,

the ships of the convoy passed through us — the ships' sides so huge and the little people at the top, calling down to us, so very small. One voice told us they daren't stop and I hoped they wouldn't because we would still be in the water when they were "fished" by the U-boat.[184]Ship after ship, and then they were gone and we were alone. The night was getting darker, the waves steeper, the breeze stronger and it seemed to be raining. The men on the rafts were singing. I recognized the commanding voice of the Gunner's Mate, Petty Officer George Grivel, a splendid man. They were singing the old favourites of the soldiers in the trenches of France and Flanders in the First World War: "Pack up your troubles in your old kit bag", "It's a long way to Tipperary" and "There's a long, long trail a-winding to the Land of My Dreams."

The hours went by, the cold became colder and now jellyfish stung my hands and arms, like torches of cold fire. When my spar gradually drifted in close to one of the floats, a Petty Officer named Locke grabbed me and held me fast against the float.[185]

At 0530, Tom Pullen "sensed rather than saw a presence nearby. Then a mass, blacker than our surroundings, materialized out of the gloom. It was the side of a ship looming over us. In Canada, the corvette *Sackville* is properly revered as the symbol of the Battle of the Atlantic. To us [survivors of *Ottawa's* sinking] then and now, there is only one corvette that will always be special. Her name is *CELANDINE*."[186]

It's helpful now to retrace *Celandine's* movements as recorded in her captain's Report of Proceedings:

[0005 September 14:]
I sighted a single white flare ahead and closed it, hoping it might be one of those for which we were searching.... I decided that I would be unjustified in stopping my ship without first sweeping around the area, which I accord-

ingly proceeded to do…. However, on closing and stopping right alongside the flares, no sign of life or survivors of any kind could be found…. I left the scene and proceeded to search away to eastward.

[Much later, about 0300:]

A tanker (*Clausina?*) was sighted stopped about 1 mile on the port beam, apparently in good trim and undamaged…. A few minutes later, many flares were sighted in the water ahead, and the sound of voices heard shortly afterwards … convinced me that they were survivors of HMCS *Ottawa*…. The night was still very dark indeed and the wind inclined to freshen. It was impossible to see many of the men in the water until we were practically on top of them and this together with the fact that the ship was constantly blowing rapidly down to leeward owing to her light condition, made the picking up of the men a very hazardous operation for them, and for us slow to a heartbreaking degree. The ship had to be manoeuvred alongside each raft and man in turn, as the majority of them had insufficient strength to attempt to swim towards us. Efforts were made to launch the sea boat, but I eventually decided to abandon this, as obviously it would be of no practical help with the sea that was running, its very limited size and its inadequate oar power.

[Then, at approximately 0400:]

In view of the great number of men still in the water, and the rather desperate tone that was becoming more apparent in their shouting, I feared that a great number would be lost before we could reach them, and signaled HMCS *St. Croix* requesting another ship be detailed to assist me. HMCS *Arvida* joined me shortly afterwards.

The rescue operation continued, and at 0535: "The last survivor that could be found [AB Alvin Wedmark] was taken aboard.… It was becoming daylight and soon a wider sweep became possible. 49 men had been picked up."

This outstanding performance becomes even more remarkable when one realizes that Lieutenant P.V. Collings, the commanding officer of *Celandine*, was just twenty-four years old!

"There were only nine left on the float when we came along side the ship [*Celandine*]," Sid Dobing says. "Lieutenant Pullen was holding onto the float [with one hand] and was towing a spar [with the other] with some survivors hanging on to it. As by this time our numbers were further reduced, the strength needed to hang on had proved for many just too much."

Celandine's Sub-Lieutenant Arnold went again and again into the water to help the wounded and weak Canadians. Dobing recalls that "during this activity, darkness was noticeably giving way to grey dawn, while the waves continued to mount, adding to our difficulties. Men nearest the ship's side, in their eagerness, scrambled out and the float, relieved of their weight, flipped. Those in the water were in danger of being swept astern under the corvette's counter and into the propeller."[187]

Collings had remained very dangerously stopped in the area for too long, and now, making sure that no one from *Ottawa* was missed, he cleared the area. At 0910: "On instructions from HMCS *St. Croix*, I took HMCS *Arvida* under my orders and set course for St. John's, Newfoundland [450 miles away] at utmost speed, both ships being very short of fuel, food and medical supplies."

Roe Skillen remembers that "all of a sudden, the dark form of a ship appeared out of the darkness" and he knew that help had come.

> God had answered my prayer. It was the corvette HMS *Celandine* and I could see the scrambling net hung over the side. There was still a heavy sea running and the Carley float was tossing. To get aboard, hitting that net at the right time was uppermost in my mind. The first attempt was a miss. As the *Celandine* rolled to port and the net was close, I grabbed it as close to the gunwale as I could. I hung on and, as I did, hands reached out and pulled me aboard. Rolling myself over, I looked into the eyes of Pat Riches,

an English sailor who I had befriended in St. John's on leave the previous Christmas. It was at this point that I discovered that I had no feeling in my legs. The crew carried me below and covered me with blankets to stop the shivering. The Skipper broke out the rum and I think that helped to save our lives. We reached St. John's in two days. I was taken to the RCNH and in the end I lost my right leg and suffered wounds to my left leg. I spent the next 3½ months there recuperating. God must have been listening that night in 1942. He has given me more than 60 years to be grateful and I thank Him for that.[188]

Edward Fox floated along for five hours, alone, clinging to a spar and supported by his bulky life jacket. Like so many others, he was stung repeatedly by jellyfish, until finally at 0500 (or thereabouts), he was picked out of the water by welcome hands on *Celandine*. The ship's Yorkshire "tiffy" (sick berth attendant) declared loudly when he broke his suturing needle in two as he began repairing Fox's wound, "Tha's got hide like a rhinoceros, lad." When *Celandine* docked in St. John's, Ed Fox was taken off immediately to the RCN Hospital there, where his extensive laceration could be re-sutured and he could recuperate for the next six weeks.

In addition to their suffering from the cold and the fuel oil that covered many of them, some of Sid Dobing's crewmates were stung by jellyfish and were in excruciating pain. However, the fuel oil turned out to be a blessing in disguise "as the jellyfish would not bother those of us who had been immersed in it."

Moe Locke still had the flashlight which all good ERAs carried and it was eventually passed to me. We decided to keep flashing the light in the hope of attracting one of the escorts looking for survivors. The night was pitch black and a heavy swell was running, making things uncomfortable and causing the raft to overturn. When it was righted, there were fewer men left and thus more room for those remaining. At 0400, we were sighted by HMS *Celandine* and rescue operations began. Scrambling nets were lowered and strong arms helped us aboard. After more than four hours adrift in the water, we were cramped and had little strength left. Some slipped from the net to their deaths just as they were approaching safety. I dropped [Moe Locke's] flashlight as I was climbing up the scrambling net. It was still shining as it sank beneath the sea.

On board, we were hustled below, oil-soaked clothing removed, given hot drinks and put into hammocks to recuperate. The next two days saw us in St. John's along with *Arvida* and *St. Croix* who were also carrying survivors. The joy of finding some of our chums on the other ships was tempered by the discovery that many others had not been picked up.

We were taken to St. John's where the injured were treated and the rest of us were sent to Halifax aboard the *Lady Rodney*. Survivors leave was granted to all of us and it was off to our homes where we recovered from the experience as best we could. The memories will never leave and those of us who did survive realize just how fortunate we were.[189]

Steve Logos remembers "when I was picked up by *Arvida*, it turned out that her Chief Stoker was from my home town, Calgary. When he found this out, he decided to look after me personally, as if I was his son. I was fed, given warm clothes and a hammock. Within 48 hours, we were in St. John's Newfoundland. We were taken up to the drill hall to be identified and to be given a complete new set of gear."[190]

The most disturbing sight for Norm Wilson that night "was when we were picked up by *Celandine*.... There were two or three who were so desperate to get on, that as the corvette rolled they got on the scrambling net on the port quarter as the ship rolled away from us ... as the ship rolled back, it rolled over them and they were lost."[191]

Eric Douglas, a DEMS gunner rescued with twenty-three of his shipmates from the torpedoed tanker *Empire Oil*, jumped into the sea from the plunging *Ottawa* without a lifebelt. He watched men who were clinging to his float just slip away exhausted and disappear into the night. He had his arm around one man for two hours until he realized the man was dead. Finally, a beam of light shone down on them. HMS *Celandine* had found them. Getting up the scrambling net to board the corvette was in itself a challenge for cold, exhausted men. A nineteen-year-old who had been near Douglas all the time on the float missed the net and was swept away to his death.[192]

Suddenly, *Celandine* arrived out of the darkness and, rolling gently, stopped alongside. Some men climbed up the scrambling net and were hauled aboard. Now it was Yogi Jenson's turn.

> I started to climb and then fell back into the water. I didn't care now what happened. If I was to drown, I was resigned. It was God's will. Strong hands from the float pushed me in toward the ship again. I reached up the net feebly and a great muscular arm reached down like the Arm of God and hauled me out of the water like a fish. I staggered clear and climbed a ladder to the upper deck. It was right over the engine room and I can still feel the warmth of that deck. Dripping wet, covered in oil, totally exhausted and half frozen, yet wonderfully contented. I had to urinate, so I just did it, like a baby in diapers. When I entered the wardroom, there was our Leading Steward Barriault who came forward and said, as if nothing unusual had happened: "Good Evening, Sir, would you like a cup of tea?" So I replied, "Good Evening, Barriault, that would be very nice, thank you." And then I had a cup of delicious, wonderful hot tea.[193]

The death tally was heart-rending. Five officers and 109 men of *Ottawa's* complement were lost. Larry Rutherford was gone, and so was George Hendry. Only sixty-nine men were rescued by *Celandine* and *Arvida.* Of the twenty-four men from the torpedoed *Empire Oil* who were rescued by *Ottawa*, DEMS gunner Eric Douglas was one of only four survivors. It had indeed been an awful night.

"The Most Commendable
Devotion to Duty"

At 1352 hours of September 15, 1942, HMS *Celandine*, with HMCS *Arvida* in close company, passed Fort Amherst at the entrance to the harbour of St. John's, Newfoundland, and docked after a rapid but uneventful passage. Both ships were very low on fuel, food, and medical supplies. *Celandine* had picked up forty-nine of *Ottawa's* survivors, including Jenson, Pullen, Lloyd Jones, Skillen, Dobing, Underhill, Fox, Johnson, Barriault, and Eric Douglas, the Royal Artillery DEMS gunner rescued from the torpedoed *Empire Oil*. *Arvida* had picked up twenty-one of her crew including Steve Logos and four seamen and DEMS gunners from *Empire Oil*.[194] Jenson recalls,

> When we arrived at St. John's, we were housed in the service quarters at Buckmaster's Field and were given civilian clothing by the Red Cross. I had an ill-fitting brown tweed jacket and flannel trousers and felt like a tramp. I am not complaining, happy as I was (and am) to be alive. The jellyfish stings had made my hands itchy, red and swollen, and for weeks, I smelled and tasted fuel oil. It seemed to have got into all the pores of my skin. I submitted a claim

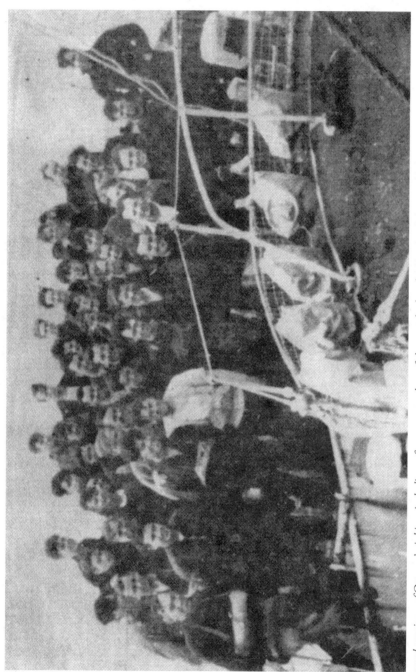

The rescued survivors of Ottawa's sinking, including a few crew members of the torpedoed tanker Empire Oil, *assembled on the quarterdeck of HMS* Celandine *on arrival in St. John's harbour, September 16, 1942. (Maritime Command Trident newspaper, May 31, 1971.)*

for the loss of all my possessions and carefully made it double what it actually was, it being my previous experience that I would receive exactly half of what I claimed. In due course, exactly half my claim was approved.[195]

Steve Logos is still bitter today about the lack of concern shown for the welfare of the surviving members of *Ottawa*'s lower deck:

All the officers were in a group by themselves and the so-called lower deck ratings were in a group by themselves. Not one of the officers walked over to greet us and to ask how we were. I would imagine that our good doctor George Hendry was up there in Heaven shaking his head that not one of our officers made a move to go over to the lower deck survivors. At that particular time, our [naval]

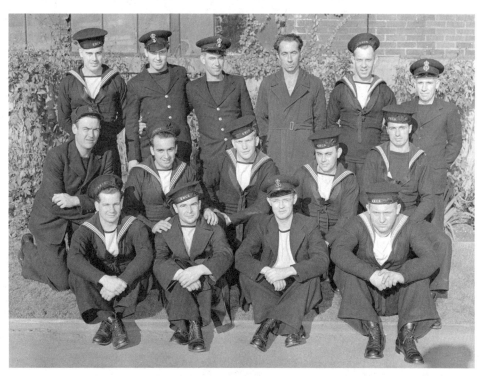

Ratings from Ontario who survived the sinking of HMCS Ottawa: Buckmaster's Field, St. John's, Newfoundland, on September 24, 1942. (Credit: Library and Archives Canada PA-204607.)

society was based on the caste system. To become an officer, your family had to have some stature or position in society which included wealth. This was really a "hand me down" from British society.[196]

They whisked Roe Skillen off *Celandine* on a stretcher and took him straight to the RCN Hospital in St. John's. After the crushing stanchion injury he had barely escaped from, followed by five hours' exposure to the cold North Atlantic, both Skillen's legs were numb from mid-thigh down and were blue-purple in colour. He couldn't feel a thing. The doctors made a diagnosis of arterial thrombosis and packed both of Roe's legs in ice in an attempt to restore the circulation. A healthy pink colour returned to his left leg but the right was beyond recovery. From above the knee it had turned an ominous mottled brown colour. Gangrene had set in, and an immediate mid-thigh amputation was the only course. Edward Fox, the ASDIC rating with the long laceration down his chest wall and trunk, had to be transferred to the Naval Hospital as well to have some secondary suturing done before being sent back to Halifax.

Except for Skillen and Fox, all of *Ottawa's* rescued seamen, including Logos, Dobing, Underhill, Soles, Johnson, and Barriault, were kept at Buckmaster's Field for a week, issued new uniforms, and then transferred to Halifax on the former Canadian National passenger steamer *Lady Rodney.* There they were given thirty days' survivor's leave in preparation for new sea postings. Eric Douglas, the lone *Empire Oil* survivor rescued from *Ottawa*, was told he wasn't fit for sea duty and was put behind a desk for the next eleven months. He didn't see any of his fellow survivors again until 1996, when he was invited back to Canada for the commissioning of the fourth *Ottawa*.

The awful news of *Ottawa's* loss was delayed by only a few days. The *Toronto Evening Telegram* for Monday, September 21, 1942, declared, "DESTROYER SUNK, 113 LOST. 12 TORONTO MEN MISSING." Around a photograph of their ship, there were heart-rending pictures of twenty-two young sailors and officers who had died.

The *Victoria Daily Times* for Monday, September 21, 1942, read, "HMCS *OTTAWA* TORPEDOED, 113 LOST." The title "*OTTAWA's* HONOUR ROLL" headed the official RCN casualty list. Then, just like in the *Telegram*, there was a photograph of the ship and pictures of four "LOCAL BOYS MISSING FROM CANADIAN DESTROYER."

Then there were the poignant tributes to George Hendry. The *Toronto Daily Star* for Tuesday, September 22, 1942, read, "SURGEON-LT. HENDRY MISSING ON *OTTAWA*. ILL-FATED TRIP WAS TO BE HIS LAST FOR SOME TIME. Returning from what was expected to be his last trip at sea for some time, Surgeon-Lieut. George A. Hendry is listed among the casualties of the Canadian destroyer *Ottawa*. He is reported 'missing, believed killed', but his family hope he is safe."

The inevitable dreaded casualty list was published in all the papers.[197] The lost 114 of *Ottawa*'s complement were there in stark relief: Hendry, Rutherford, MacMillan, Sub-Lieutenant Donald Wilson (who'd gone below to salvage the ship's confidential books in spite of Yogi Jenson's pleading), Electrician William Hobbis (who rigged the operating room lights for both operations), Stoker Petty Officer Frank Morrison (who'd just come on duty when the second torpedo struck boiler room no. 2), and the other stoker Morrison (Harry, from Toronto), Cliff Riches, young Jimmy Gibb, and, of course, Pooch Bucheski, the appendectomy patient.

September 6 to 13, 1942, was a bad week for the Royal Canadian Navy. Before *Ottawa* was lost, U-boats torpedoed and sank two more of its ships in the St. Lawrence River with heavy loss of life.

On September 6, 1942, HMCS *Raccoon*, a converted yacht of 377 tons, assigned to the Gulf Escort Force, along with the corvette *Arrowhead*, the minesweeper-escort *Truro*, and two Fairmile launches, was shepherding the eight ships of convoy QS 33 (Quebec-Sydney) past Father Point on the south shore of the river. At 2110, the Greek freighter *Aeas*, of 4,700 tons, was torpedoed by the U-165 and sank quickly. *Arrowhead* altered back and, searching the area by starshell illumination, managed to make out the dim silhouette of *Raccoon*. At 0010, two explosions were heard to the rear of the convoy and then nothing more. Again *Arrowhead* put about and swept around in the pitch black of the night but nothing was seen or heard of *Raccoon* again. Much later, U-165's shot report (*schussmeldung*) indicated that two torpedoes had struck the little ship and she was literally obliterated. There were no survivors from a complement of four officers and thirty-three ratings. Some weeks later, the body of Sub-Lieutenant Russ McConnell, an outstanding McGill University athlete before the war, along with a small piece of wooden bridge structure and a lifesaver, was all that was ever found of the little *Raccoon*.

Five days later, on September 11, 1942, the corvette *Charlottetown* was torpedoed by U-517 on the north side of the St. Lawrence, as she was returning to Gaspé after escorting the Sydney-to-Quebec convoy SQ 35 to Rimouski. The ship was struck by two torpedoes in rapid succession at 0800 and sank in three minutes. There had been no warning of the presence of a submarine, as ASDIC 's efficiency was drastically reduced by the mix of salt and fresh water in that area of the St. Lawrence near the mouth of the Saguenay River. Six of the nine crew members lost (including the captain, Lieutenant J.W. Bonner) were killed in the water by dreadful abdominal immersion injuries caused by the ship's depth charges exploding as she sank. It had all been so quick that there had been no time to ditch the primers on the depth charges.

In a sad little letter, George's mother wrote to Betty Summers:

> You have been in my thoughts so constantly and I can't get alone at the phone, since the relatives are here all the time. I want you to know how I suffered with you. I know what you meant to George and I know what a tragedy this is for both of us.
>
> But Betty dear, you have life before you and your sorrow will be lessened by time. I know that the sharp edges are removed, otherwise we couldn't carry on at all. Your friends are thinking and praying for you as they are for me. Just now I feel as if there was nothing left but we have to be brave as George would have us be. Henry Swan said in a card I received this morning "George never showed his feelings and we must not let him down now"....
>
> "Grief being private must be borne alone although I cannot share your sorrow (I certainly can because <u>I know how you have been cheated out of your happiness</u>) still anguished tears are mingled with my own. I walk unseen beside you up the hill". That little poem came to me in a

note this morning and I thought it might help. God help us both to bear this sorrow, under such terrible conditions.

Lovingly, his mother

Elizabeth Hendry

Saturday, September 26

On November 1, 1942, All Saints' Day, Rev. Dr. W.H. Sedgewick, the minister at Westminster Central United Church on Bloor Street East in Toronto, proclaimed to the congregation that "it is a happy coincidence that brings to our service this morning the superintendents, doctors, nurses and friends of Toronto General Hospital … come to pay their tribute of respect and affection to one who was at once a member of the staff of the Hospital and a son of this church — Surgeon Lieutenant George Ainslie Hendry." Elizabeth Hendry sat in front with her nieces, Carol Hendry and Edith Hendry Will. Sitting by herself in a pew opposite this mighty company was Betty Summers. Arthur Squires's wife, Miriam, remembers that she saw Betty sitting alone at the memorial service.

The disturbing story of George Hendry's entrapment and subsequent escape had been so suppressed by Toronto General Hospital society that very few people at the hospital knew of George's relationship with Betty Summers. Frank Shipp, Henry Swan, and Arthur Squires were already overseas before George had met Betty. Even now, the surviving members of Jean Matthews's TGH nursing class of 1938 are completely unaware of Betty Summers's existence.

Certainly, Jean Matthews Hendry was not there in the church. She had been back home in Calgary many months before *Ottawa* and George were lost. There had been a frozen silence in the corridors of the TGH about the details of Jean's fabrication, entrapment, and deception. This was a skeleton exclusively in the TGH closet. George and Jean were TGH; Betty Summers was Women's College, and an outsider, if indeed she existed at all in the minds of the people just across College Street. There was a very straightforward explanation for Betty's anonymity: George Hendry was a very private person and so was Betty Summers.

On October 24, 1942, Dr. Ralph Will, serving as a medical officer with a Canadian Army Ordinance Unit in England, wrote to my father:

Dear Jimmy,

We all have been greatly shocked over George's loss.... Edith [Ralph Will's wife and Carol Hendry Duffus's sister] has written of continuing hopes, but one can hardly see how that is possible.

There is no doubt that George was one of the finest chaps that many of us have known; in fact, I can't remember hearing anyone say anything against him. When he was over in August, he looked up his friends, particularly at the 15th General, came down to find me with Mel Watson and I spent the rest of the day with him at Mel's unit. That tragic marriage or any other misjudgment doesn't change our attitude but it was difficult for those closest to him....

(sgd)."Ralph E. Will"

Shortly after *Celandine* and *Arvida* docked with the sixty-nine rescued members of *Ottawa*'s crew, a Board of Inquiry was convened in the office of the Captain (D) Newfoundland, Captain E.R. Mainguy, RCN, in the Old Knights of Columbus Building on Queen Street in St. John's. The board was charged with looking into "the circumstances attending the loss of HMCS *Ottawa* on Sunday, 13 September 1942." Lieutenant T.C. Pullen and Sub-Lieutenant L.B. Jenson were called to appear before the board. "During the inquiry into the loss of the *Ottawa*," Steve Logos recalls with some bitterness, "not one of the 'lower deck', petty officers or ratings, was called."[198]

Yogi Jenson remembers that "we appeared individually before the Board of Inquiry. Commander 'Scarface' Holmes (who was not officially a part of the inquiry) asked me when the first torpedo hit. I replied 'at 1103' or so and received quite a blast for not saying '2303'."[199]

The board's findings and recommendations were duly reported on September 20, 1942, in appropriately terse service language. The full text of the findings of the Board of Inquiry is provided in Appendix D. Included was a commendation to the company of HMCS *Ottawa*:

The ship was efficient and well organized as is shown by the evidence that everybody knew and carried out their duties in the emergency.

The morale of the ship's company throughout was magnificent.

The Board wishes to draw special attention to the commendable devotion to duty (shown in evidence) of the following officers and men:-

The Commanding Officer, Acting Lieutenant-Commander Clark A. Rutherford, RCN and the Medical Officer, Surgeon Lieutenant George A. Hendry, RCNVR. These officers lost their lives largely through exhaustion caused by little or no rest for some days previously. Also to Sub-Lieutenant L.B. Jenson who, for a young officer, displayed considerable initiative and powers of command. [Also to:]

Acting Gunner (T) L.I. Jones
Petty Officer G.Q. Grivel
Leading Stoker M.A. McLeod
Sub-Lieutenant Arnold of HMS *Celandine.*

After the inquiry came the postmortems.[200] Captain (D) for Newfoundland, Captain E.R. "Rollo" Mainguy, congratulated the C-4 escort group for a job well done on their arrival in St. John's. The Flag Officer Newfoundland Force (FONF) Rear Admiral L.W. Murray laid the blame for the loss of seven merchant ships and particularly of *Ottawa* on the lack of the superior Type 271 radar in five of six of the escort vessels; the Royal Navy corvette *Celandine* was the only ship so equipped and its set was unserviceable for most of the trip.

On the other hand, the representatives of the Admiralty, Commander Howard-Johnston and Captain Ravenhill, were scathing in their criticism of C-4's SOE, Lieutenant Commander Dobson, for his perceived mismanagement of his escort vessels, frittering away essential convoy coverage by detailing them to drop way back to sink torpedoed merchant ships, and accused the senior Canadian naval officers, Mainguy and Murray, of outright incompetence. Ravenhill was particularly scornful that neither officer had "the remotest idea of what was expected of them" and dismissed the situation as a "complete muddle."[201]

This rant allowed the Admiralty to neatly sidestep its undeniably major responsibility by refusing any cooperation with the Canadian government, the National Research Council in Ottawa, or the Royal Canadian Navy in the development or provision of the far more advanced Type 271 radar. In fact, nowhere in the British critique of the shortcomings of C-4 and the Royal Canadian Navy was there a single reference to this glaring oversight.

The day after the exhausted remainder of C-4 escort force docked in St. John's (September 16), Rear Admiral Leonard Murray, the outgoing flag officer Newfoundland Force, sent a strongly worded request to NSHQ in Ottawa that all MOEF escort be pushed to the head of the queue for the fitting of 271 radar. On October 1, 1942, the naval staff, moving with uncharacteristic swiftness, gave its approval in principle for the removal of gunnery rangefinders in River class destroyers and their replacement with the superior anti-submarine radar equipment.

However, it was not until November 24, 1942, that the director of naval construction at NSHQ finally stated in a memorandum concerning the recommendations of the Board of Inquiry into the loss of HMCS *Ottawa* that RDF Type 271 should be fitted to all convoy escorts as quickly as the equipment was available and the ships were available for fitting of same.

This directive applied as well to the fitting of HF/DF type FH3 radio-triangulation equipment ("Huff-Duff") in all destroyers.

Sadly, these long overdue provisions were not made soon enough. In the first week of November, Convoy SC 107 escorted by C-4 lost nine ships (seven in one day) in mid-Atlantic to the seventeen U-boats of *Gruppe Veilchen*.

Only two of six escorts had 271 radar, *Restigouche* (SOE; Lieutenant-Commander D.W. Piers, RCN) and *Celandine*, and, just as it had happened with ON 127 in September, *Celandine*'s set broke down for most of the battle. If this weren't enough, there was only one serviceable HF/DF (in *Restigouche*), when this method of anti-submarine tracking requires two units to be functional.

Because of all too characteristic service stagnation, most Canadian escort warships weren't fitted with 271 radar and HF/DF until well into the spring of 1943.

After she had torpedoed and sunk *Ottawa*, U-91 was attacked with depth charges unsuccessfully (possibly by *St. Croix*) and managed to slip away in the dark.[202] Later on this patrol, she sank a seven-thousand-ton ship. On October 6, 1942, she arrived at Brest, where she joined the 9th U-boat Flotilla. U-91's third patrol was Heinz Walkerling's last. On February 11, 1943, she sailed to a station in the North Atlantic and there she sank four merchant ships totalling twenty-nine thousand tons.

With Kapitän-Leutnant Heinz Hungershausen in command, U-91 sailed from Brest on her sixth and last patrol on January 25, 1944, as part of a fifteen–U-boat wolf pack. After nearly a month of seeing nothing at all, she was suddenly attacked on the surface at 2330 of February 25, 1944, by aircraft and by three Royal Navy destroyers, *Affleck*, *Gore*, and *Gould*. Submerging deeply to 200 metres (656 feet), she was severely damaged by the third pattern of depth charges dropped. Her ballast tanks were blown and she shot to the surface. The boat was finally sunk by gunfire and thirty-seven of her company were lost. Hungershausen and fifteen others were rescued.

Unlike more than twenty-nine thousand German submariners, Kapitän-Leutnant Heinz Walkerling survived the war and never went to sea again. In 1946, he went into the banking business and eventually became the director of a bank in Mülheim in the Ruhr. Yogi Jenson contacted him in 1970 when gathering material for a book on the loss of the *Ottawa*, but they never met.

At 2115 hours of September 20, 1943, U-305 (under the command of Kapitän-Leutnant Rudolph Bahr) blew the stern off HMCS *St. Croix* with one of the new *Zaunkönig*[203] acoustic torpedoes, but the old ship managed to stay afloat. An hour later, however, another of these new torpedoes cut her in two and she sank in three minutes. Seventy-six ratings and five officers of *St. Croix* (including the captain, Lieutenant Commander A.H. Dobson) were rescued at dawn by the corvette HMS *Itchen* after a long night in the water.[204]

Forty hours later, U-666 fired two of the acoustic torpedoes. One missed HMS *Morden* but the other struck *Itchen* midships in a huge explosion. She rolled over and sank in less than a minute. In the end, Stoker William Fisher of *St. Croix* and two ratings from *Itchen* were all who remained of nearly four hundred men of the two ships' companies. Andrew Hedley Dobson was gone, as was Surgeon Lieutenant William Lyon Mackenzie King, the namesake and nephew of Canada's wartime prime minister. He and George Hendry were the only members of the staff of the Toronto General Hospital to be killed in action during the Second World War. William Fisher, *St. Croix*'s lone survivor, lived to age eighty-one in Alberta and died of a heart attack in 2001.

Both George Hendry and Larry Rutherford were Mentioned in Despatches posthumously.[205] This award was gazetted on January 1, 1943.

Hendry's citation read as follows: "Whilst serving in one of HMC Destroyers in the North Atlantic, the late Surgeon Lieutenant George Ainslie Hendry performed outstanding surgical work aboard his ship, and displayed at all times the most commendable devotion to duty."

Rutherford's citation read as follows: "In command of one of HMC Destroyers in the North Atlantic, the late Acting Lieutenant-Commander Clark Anderson Rutherford displayed outstanding zeal and wholehearted devotion to duty, worthy of the best traditions of the Royal Canadian Navy."

In an old file squirrelled away somewhere in the bowels of the Department of National Defence, there is one of those predictably impersonal forms entitled "Accounts of Men Discharged ('whether discharged on shore, D.D., or run')." In it, the two RCN paymasters "certify that we have every reason to believe that the above account contains a true statement of all wages, Effects, and other Credits or Debts (for 'Hendry, G.A., Surgeon Lieutenant, RCNVR') on the ledger of ... H.M.C.S. 'Ottawa' ... amounting to a net balance of Two Hundred and thirty six dollars Ninety four cents. Dated on board H.M.C.S. ... "Avalon" ... at ... St. John's, Newfoundland ... this ... Thirteenth ... day of ... November ... 1942."

And that was all his country said it owed the late George Ainslie Hendry "who D.D. ['discharged dead'] ... on the 13th September ... 1942."

Sid Dobing went up to Trois-Rivières on his survivor's leave to see young Jimmy Gibb's mother:

> Jimmy Gibb joined the *Ottawa* sometime in 1942 and was in the torpedomen's mess, as he had hopes of becoming a Seaman Torpedoman. He was 19 at the time and the only son who retained some of his English accent. His parents had moved to Canada in the 30s, when Jimmy was quite young. He and I became good friends,

[he was] a likable, happy-go-lucky chap with a smile on his face, a very good messmate.

I was not with Jimmy when the ship sank and didn't know, until all of us who had survived met in St. John's and inquiries confirmed, that he had been lost. When I was on survivor's leave, I wrote to his parents in Three Rivers, Quebec to express my condolences and to tell them of our friendship. I received a reply almost immediately from Mrs. Gibb who asked if I could possibly stop over on my return from leave and spend some time with them. I agreed and they met me in Montreal and we drove to Three Rivers.

Mrs. Gibb asked me to give them any details that I thought of what had happened that night, particularly in connection with their son. She also asked if I could tell her just what time the ship had been sunk and she said that she had a reason for asking the question. I told her that we had been hit just after 2300 and that the second torpedo had struck about 20 minutes later and that we had abandoned ship right after that. She then told me the reason for the question.

Apparently that evening, Mr. and Mrs. Gibb were having a quiet evening at home when Jimmy's dog, Skipper, started to whine. Mr. Gibb let him out and within a few minutes he whined to be let in. Another few minutes and he wanted to go out again and then back in. This behavior was repeated another couple of times and then Mrs. Gibb said to her husband that Jimmy was in trouble. Her husband said that she was probably imagining things, trying to reassure her by saying that the dog probably was not well. We then compared times of incidence with the dog and the sinking of the *Ottawa* and allowing for the difference in time zones, Skipper had whined and fussed during the period that Jimmy must have been in the water. This convinced Mrs. Gibb that the dog sensed that his master was in trouble and that it wasn't until Jimmy died that Skipper stopped this odd behavior. Skeptics will say that it was just a coincidence, but I like to think that Mrs. Gibb was right when she said that the dog knew that Jimmy was in trouble.[206]

Before the onset of the Second World War, Michael Barriault sailed with some boys from the Bay of Islands region in Newfoundland, including his good friend Frank Morrison. This group of boys was on board the SS *Humber Arm* when she was torpedoed off the coast of Ireland on July 8, 1940. Barriault went back to Newfoundland to work until he joined the Royal Canadian Navy. He was posted to HMCS *Ottawa*, where he again met his friend Frank Morrison, who had been on the *Ottawa* for some time and was now a petty officer stoker. On the night that the *Ottawa* was sunk, Morrison relieved his mate in the engine room, just before the first torpedo struck. The second torpedo struck the *Ottawa* in the boiler room area. The destroyer heeled over and began to sink. Barriault knew full well that his friend didn't have a chance. One of the most difficult things that Michael Barriault ever had to do was to visit Frank Morrison's mother after he was lost.

On September 20, immediately after appearing before the Board of Inquiry looking into the sinking of the *Ottawa*, Tom Pullen returned home to Toronto to marry Betty Wheelright, his sweetheart from high school days before he had gone overseas for officer training in 1936. In anticipation of this, he'd had a new uniform made in London but of course it had been lost when *Ottawa* sank. So he had to have another made quickly in Toronto.

Betty and Tom were married on Wednesday, September 30, 1942, in St. Simon's Church on Bloor Street East. They used their honeymoon to visit the families of the Toronto and Peterborough men lost in *Ottawa*, and Tom went around to the Hendry family home to sit with George's mother.

Yogi Jenson went home to Calgary on his survivor's leave, and while there he went around to express his condolences to Jean Hendry. He had just finished introducing himself when she turned away without uttering a word and closed the door, leaving Jenson standing on the stoop, astonished. Later, Yogi decided that Jean must have been sure that George Hendry had confided her deception to him. However, being the very private person that he was, George told no one of his humiliation, not even Yogi. So, I think we have to conclude that Jean's puzzling performance at the door reflected not only grief but shame and guilt as well.

Epilogue:
A Closed Book

$\mathcal{T}$he war in Europe ended with the unconditional surrender of German armed forces on May 8, 1945. The Battle of the Atlantic ("the Longest Battle") had been won but at an enormous cost to both sides. U-boats of the *Reichsmarine* sank 13.5 million deadweight tons of Allied merchant shipping, 2,603 ships with the loss of 30,000 seamen. Of 40,000 German submariners, nearly 30,000 were lost at sea. The ships of the Royal Canadian Navy sank 47 German U-boats and two Italian submarines, but at a cost of 24 warships and nearly 1,800 officers and men.

What of all those who loved George Hendry and grieved for him, those left behind in Toronto and those far away? What became of his surviving shipmates from *Ottawa* who felt his loss so keenly?

On June 11, 1948, Elizabeth Robertson Hendry died. Carol Hendry Duffus says her aunt Bessie died of a broken heart. It was rather like a Greek tragedy. All her men were gone, her husband, Will, and her two boys, Jack and George. She was left alone with her memories in a small upper duplex at 1393 Avenue Road in North Toronto. She wrote to Betty Summers (now in the RCN Nursing Service in Sydney, Nova Scotia) on March 23, 1945:

There is an article in the Canadian Medical Association Journal on ethical conduct and the concluding paragraph called "The Long Shadows" seems to be a tribute to Dr. Hendry, Jack and George; beautifully written.[207] I shouldn't keep George as much in your mind, but he is in mine and naturally I talk about him…. I copied the article and am sending it to you…. This may not have any one in mind — but the two sons [in the article] are exceptional, and make me think of my boys….

Well, that's a sad note to send on, but … I know you feel that, in spite of everything, your love and affection were not misplaced … in spite of the sorrow it has caused … you and those who loved him as we did. Well Dear, write when you can and may the future bring you happiness in spite of everything.

Lovingly,

Bessie Hendry

Elizabeth Hendry left the University of Toronto an endowment of $4,500 to establish the Hendry Memorial Scholarship:

… in memory of the late Professor Emeritus W.B. Hendry; the late William John Hendry who graduated from the University of Toronto as Gold Medallist in Medicine in 1933 and who died in 1934 at Baltimore, while engaged in experimental research at the Carnegie Institution of Washington; and the late Surgeon Lieutenant George Ainslie Hendry, MD 1935, who died on active service in 1942. The award is made annually to an undergraduate medical student of the final year, who, in the opinion of the Chair of the Department of Obstetrics and Gynaecology, is most worthy of the award. The following considerations are to be the basis of the award: character, sportsmanship and scholastic attainment.

The Hendry Memorial Scholarship is offered to this day at the University of Toronto.

After his survivor's leave following the loss of *Ottawa*, newly promoted Lieutenant L.B. "Yogi" Jenson, RCN, became at age twenty-one the youngest first lieutenant (of the destroyer HMCS *Niagara*) in the history of the Royal Canadian Navy, and then, at age twenty-two, its youngest captain (briefly during her commissioning trials of the corvette HMCS *Long Branch*). Then early in 1944, he was appointed first lieutenant of the destroyer *Algonquin*, whose captain was Lieutenant Commander D.W. "Debby" Piers, DSC, RCN, and whose navigation officer was Lieutenant R.M. "Dick" Steele, RCNVR. *Algonquin* was in the van of the escorting ships at the D-Day landings on Juno Beach in Normandy and then took part in raids on German ships, including the huge battleship *Tirpitz*.

For two years (1945 and 1946) as senior term lieutenant at the Royal Canadian Naval College, Royal Roads, Yogi taught future admirals and senior naval officers, several of whom became lifelong friends. Later as Commander L.B. Jenson, RCN, he commanded the destroyers *Crusader* and *Micmac*, the frigate *Fort Erie*, and the Seventh Escort Squadron.

Yogi retired from the navy in 1964, just before Paul Hellyer's homogenization of the Canadian armed forces, and settled in Queensland, down the shore from the Head of St. Margaret's Bay, Nova Scotia, with his wonderful wife, Alma. Now he employed his very considerable talent as a naval artist, writing and illustrating sixteen books on the great fishing schooners, old Halifax waterfront buildings, scenes of rural Nova Scotia, and, of course, his epic autobiography, *Tin Hats, Oilskins and Seaboots*. As chairman of the advisory council of the Maritime Museum, he spearheaded the acquisition of HMCS *Sackville*, the last remaining corvette from the Second World War, as a floating memorial to those who fought and won the Battle of the Atlantic. In spring 2004, Latham B. Jenson was awarded the Order of Canada for these services to our maritime heritage.

Yogi survived two major cardiac surgeries, and despite repeated bouts of heart failure right up to the last months of his life, he joined his old friends retired Rear Admiral Desmond W. "Debby" Piers, DSC, RCN, and retired Captain (N) R.M. "Dick" Steele, DSC, RCN, as well as several of his old students from Royal Roads days for lunch down the road in Bridgewater, Nova Scotia.

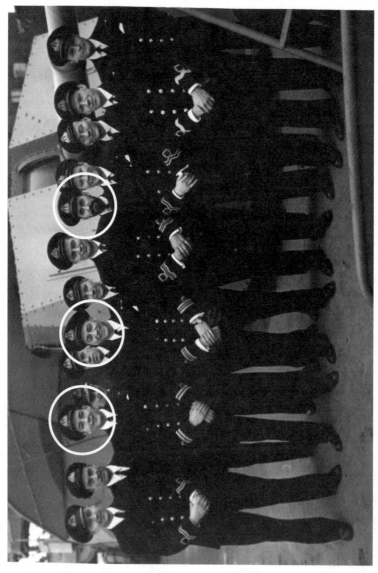

The officers of HMCS Algonquin, spring 1944: Lieutenant L.B. "Yogi" Jenson, RCN (First Lieutenant); Lieutenant Commander D.W. "Debby" Piers, RCN (Captain); Lieutenant R.M. "Dick" Steele, RCNVR (Navigator).

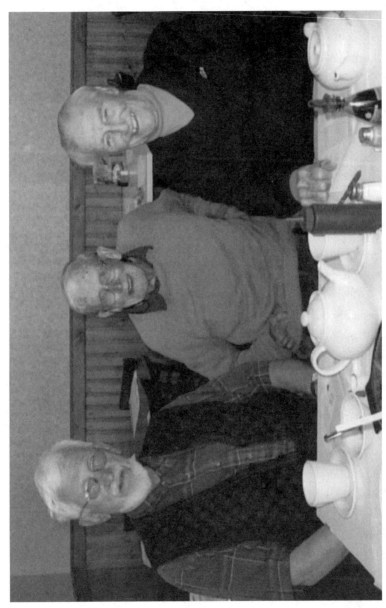

"Hearts of Oak": Dick Steele, Yogi Jenson, and Debby Piers met for lunch every Tuesday at Bridgewater, Nova Scotia. This photograph was taken in February 2004, exactly sixty years after the photo opposite. (Courtesy of Alma Jenson.)

Yogi lost his last battle against heart failure and pneumonia on the night of December 29, 2004. As he wished, half his ashes were committed to the sea at 44° 37″N, 63° 32″W on May 26, 2005. The remainder were scattered in the woods near his home.

I wrote in his obituary on April 12, 2005: "This remarkable man loved life, had a strong faith, a kindly tolerance of his own and other peoples' foibles, and a great sense of humour. He was the best of shipmates, a gentle man and a gentleman. As Dick Steele, his old friend and fellow officer on *Algonquin* said: 'I thank God that I had the honour of serving with this man.'"

Yogi Jenson was, and will always be, the spirit of the old Royal Canadian Navy.

Tom Pullen returned from survivor's leave and his honeymoon to continue the classic naval career: commanding three destroyers (*Saskatchewan*, *Iroquois*, and *Huron*) and a frigate (*La Hulloise*), *Huron* again as commander Canadian destroyers Far East (1953–54), and the naval supply ship *Protector*. However, the pursuit that changed his life and that was the "happiest time" in his naval career was the command of the Arctic patrol ship/icebreaker HMCS *Labrador*, from February 1956 to December 1957.[208] Not only did he conduct extensive hydrographic and oceanographic surveys widely in Arctic waters, he also discovered a safe and easier channel for ship passage to Frobisher Bay (now Iqaluit) and led an RCN–USN naval task force that demonstrated the existence of a usable deep-water channel through the particularly treacherous Bellot Strait between the northern most tip of the North American continent and Somerset Island. This was hailed as a remarkable piece of Arctic navigation and survey work.

Captain (N) T.C. Pullen retired in 1966 at age forty-seven, and in the next twenty years he was frequently sought as a consultant, giving crucial hydrographic and navigational advice on the passage of ships like the huge American tanker *Manhattan* through sovereign Canadian Arctic waters and similar concerns relating to mineral, oil, and gas exploration and transport in the Arctic.

In 1984, he was made an Officer of the Order of Canada, and later that year "Thomas Charles Pullen, OC, CD, RCN (Ret'd), Arctic Explorer, Navigator, Surveyor, Ice Master, Author, Lecturer and Naval

Captain" was presented for the degree of Doctor of Science, *honoris causa,* at Royal Roads University, Esquimalt, British Columbia.[209]

After a short illness, Tom Pullen died in Ottawa on August 3, 1990, age seventy-one. As Graham Rowley wrote, "He had become, and to the last he remained, one of the great polar navigators."[210]

Larry and Marjorie Rutherford's only child, Robert Anderson Rutherford, was born on December 7, 1941, the "Day of Infamy" at Pearl Harbor, a scant nine months before Larry died when *Ottawa* was lost. Following in his father's footsteps, Bob Rutherford graduated from Royal Roads and Royal Military College in 1962 and progressed through several seagoing appointments as a weapons system specialist to the command of the destroyer helicopter escort *Margaree* (as Commander R.A. Rutherford) from 1978 to 1980 and on to senior staff positions with NATO in Germany and National Defence Headquarters in Ottawa. He retired from the navy in 1995 and lives in Bedford, Nova Scotia.

In early February 1943, Lieutenant Dunn Lantier, RCN, was posted to the newly commissioned Tribal class destroyer HMCS *Athabaskan.*

On August 27, 1943, Lantier was wounded when the ship was badly damaged by a glider bomb while patrolling off the Spanish coast. The ship was extensively repaired over the next four months and Dunn recovered from his injury. He was promoted to lieutenant commander on January 1, 1944, and returned to duty in *Athabaskan.* On April 29, 1944, while engaged with the 10th Destroyer Flotilla (including *Haida*) against enemy light naval forces, the ship was torpedoed by the German torpedo Boat T-24. The captain (Lieutenant Commander J.H. Stubbs, DSO, RCN) and 128 of the ship's complement were lost, and Dunn Lantier, along with eighty-two others, was taken prisoner. He spent the next year in a German POW camp outside Bremen.

After spending the first few postwar years at Staff College and in the Directorate of Naval Plans at the Department of National Defence in Ottawa, Dunn was appointed as executive officer (first lieutenant commander) to the aircraft carrier HMCS *Magnificient* in 1950–52. He was promoted to commander and appointed to command the famed destroyer HMCS *Haida* from 1952 to 1953 (Korean War). During this conflict, he was awarded the Distinguished Service Cross (DSC).

In 1960, Lantier was appointed Canadian Naval attaché in Ankara, Turkey, for three years. He retired from the navy in 1964 just as the "Hellyer Homogenization" of the armed forces was about to begin and was subsequently engaged as a senior executive with EXPO '67. Sadly, Dunn developed a very aggressive carcinoma of the oesophagus and died on December 5, 1985.

After his survivor's leave, Lloyd Jones, *Ottawa's* torpedo gunner, was posted alternately to shore establishments instructing at HMCS *Stadacona* and HMCS *Cornwallis* and then sea duty in the legendary Tribal class destroyer *Haida* and the aircraft carrier *Warrior*. He received his full commission as gunner (T) in 1944 and rose to the rank of lieutenant commander by 1954 as a torpedo anti-submarine (TAS) specialist. From 1948, he did shore duty as senior instructor and later as an administrator at HMCS *Naden* in Esquimalt and sea duty as first lieutenant of the minesweepers *New Liskeard* and *Pictou* and then commanded the destroyer *Crescent* and the minesweeper *Brockville*.

He retired from the navy in 1961 and died in Victoria on April 8, 1991.

Something more must be added to such a seemingly impersonal catalogue of this man's naval service. Dick Steele, Yogi Jenson's fellow officer in *Algonquin* in 1944, shared Yogi's warm admiration of Lloyd Jones: "He was a very fine man."

For six months following the amputation of his right leg, and after the inevitable discharge from the navy, Roe Skillen worked for two paper companies in northwestern Ontario and then became manager of the Liquor Control Board store in his hometown, Nipigon, Ontario. "I retired from that position in 1982 after 32½ years of service. Then I went fishing."[211] I had a number of delightful talks with Roe over the past few years, but I regret that I never met him — or most of the old survivors of the ship. Sadly, during the fall of 2005, he lost weight rapidly, probably due to cancer, according to his daughter. Roe died at home on January 7, 2006. He was eighty-seven.

When Alvin Underhill was posted to *Cornwallis* in 1952 as chief petty officer in charge of security, it turned out that Commander T.C. Pullen was in command of the base. When Underhill told Pullen (who didn't recognize him at first) that the last time they had been together "was hanging on to a Carley float in the North Atlantic ten years ago," Tom (as Al tells it) "just about jumped over his desk and kissed me."[212] Shortly thereafter, Tom Pullen recommended Al for a commission, and he subsequently became security inspector for the entire RCN. Retiring as a lieutenant commander in 1971, he went on to a new career as justice of the peace in the Halifax Family Court and was supervisor of that court for more than fourteen years.

Staying in the navy after the war, Sid Dobing was coxswain (and then commanded!) the *Fairmile* M 124, a wooden motor launch. Sid was then coxswain in *Athabaskan* and *Margaree*, and then retired from the navy in 1960. In retirement, he qualified as a registered social worker at the University of Victoria and worked in Veterans' Hospital Social Work until his second retirement in 1985.

Sid attended the commissioning of *Ottawa IV* in Cornwall, Ontario, in late 1996:

> There were about a dozen of us present who had survived
> the sinking of the first *Ottawa*. Among the guests was a
> Mrs. Lewis, who was a daughter of Alex MacMillan [the
> Sick Birth Attendant in first *Ottawa*] who was just three
> years old at the time of his death. I spent quite a lot of time
> with her … explaining just what her Dad had done before
> the sinking. I was glad to be able to fill her in on his … last
> duties on board *Ottawa*. Mrs. MacMillan did not remarry
> following Alex's death and had died in 1995, the year
> before [the reunion at] the commissioning ceremonies.[213]

After *Ottawa* was lost, Steve Logos rose rapidly in the ranks; by the end of the war he was a petty officer (leading torpedo operator). "I used my authority with care and considered the dignity of the other person," Steve says, reflecting his opinion of the vast social hiatus that existed between officers and men in the Royal Canadian Navy of 1942.[214]

Sometime after Leading Steward Michael Barriault served wet, cold, newly rescued Sub-Lieutenant L.B. Jenson a very welcome cup of tea on board HMS *Celandine*, he began a long career as chief steward and mess manager in four ships and on the personal staff of Vice-Admiral H.T.W. Grant, the chief of the naval staff in Ottawa. One of the highlights of his service career was his appointment as chief steward in the aircraft carrier

Magnificent during the coronation of Queen Elizabeth II in 1953. After his retirement from the navy in 1965, he was club manager for the Bowater Paper Mill Employees Union in Cornerbrook for another twenty-two years. Michael Barriault died on January 23, 2004.

Eric Douglas, the only "double survivor" of *Empire Oil* and *Ottawa* to be rescued by *Celandine* after a long night in the dark, cold Atlantic, was put behind a desk until he was finally discharged home to England in 1946. He returned to his trade as a fabric dyer in Nottingham and saw no more of his fellow survivors until September 1996, when he and his wife were suddenly invited to attend the commissioning of the new patrol frigate *Ottawa IV* in Cornwall, Ontario.

He has one rather practical memory of September 13–14, 1942: "While I was in the water, I remembered thinking that if I was finished here, I shan't know who won the war."[215]

After he was discharged from the navy as a leading stoker (with petty officer qualification), George Johnson completed the apprenticeship training as a plumber that he had started before the war and began a successful business in that trade in Burlington, Ontario. For his long-time community leadership in the Scouting movement, he was named Burlington's "Citizen of the Year" in 1963. George retired in 1991 to Sundridge, Ontario. Sadly, he died suddenly on November 30, 2006, while driving home after mailing Christmas cards to friends.

Edward Fox finished the war as a lieutenant in the RCNVR and went on to graduate in chemical engineering from the University of Toronto in 1949. His professional career involved work in environmental water management. In retirement at age eighty-four and living in East Toronto, Ed developed amyotrophic lateral sclerosis (Lou Gehrig's disease) and died from its complications on January 9, 2004.

Coming back on the train to Halifax in the fall of 1942 following his survivor's leave after the sinking of *Ottawa*, Terry Terrabassi met Mildred, the girl he would marry in April 1943. He was drafted to the corvette HMCS *Edmonston* as a radar operator for nine months, and then, after an advanced radar course, he was posted to the cruiser HMCS *Uganda* and served the rest of the war in her.

After the war, he worked in Detroit, Michigan, in his old trade as a butcher and then as a meat market manager. He retired in 1985 and now lives with his family in Dallas, Texas. His proud daughter Nancy writes, "Terry loves his family. He is a fabulous husband, father, grandfather and great-grandfather. My Dad used to tell us that God must have had a plan for him because he was not married and did not have any family to speak of when he was saved."[216]

Norm Wilson became a telecommunications manager after the war, and this job took him first to the Dominican Republic, then to Venezuela, Surinam, United States, South Africa, and back to the Dominican Republic for thirteen years. He retired to the United States and finally returned to Canada three years ago to settle down with his wife, Louise, in Bowser, B.C., on Vancouver Island. Norm, now eighty-five, is fit and promises to live to one hundred!

Now, sadly, there are only six survivors of *Ottawa's* sinking living in 2007: Logos, Dobing, Underhill, Terrabassi, Wilson, and Douglas, the rescued *Empire Oil* gunner.

Frank Shipp, George Hendry's best friend, went overseas in 1940 as a surgeon with the 15th Canadian General Hospital at Bramshott in England. In late 1943, he was posted to a front-line, *MASH* type surgical unit in Italy. Frank finished the war as a lieutenant colonel and was awarded the OBE for his military service.

Frank practised orthopaedic surgery for thirty-five years, first in Boston at the Lahey Clinic, the Massachusetts General, and Peter Bent Brigham hospitals, and then from 1951 in four Bay Area hospitals in the city of Richmond just outside San Francisco. Frank held an appointment as a clinical professor of surgery at the University of California at San Francisco.

Frank retired from active practice in 1982, and two years later he became incapacitated with a dementia similar to Alzheimer's disease. Very sadly, one evening in December 1985, he walked out of his long-term care facility in a confused state and wandered off in the dark. He was found two days later. He had collapsed in a ditch and had died of hypothermia. He was seventy-three.

Just days before *Ottawa's* last convoy run out of Northern Ireland, George Hendry had a very fast trip on an RAF "sked run" to London to lunch with Henry (Hank) Swan on his way down to Bramshott to visit with Frank Shipp at 15 Canadian General Hospital. After the war, Hank Swan went into general practice in Burk's Falls and Barrie, Ontario, where he died at age eighty-eight in 1999.

Arthur Squires became a consultant haematologist at the Toronto General Hospital, and then in 1960 he went to the Wellesley Hospital as physician-in-chief. He taught clinical microscopy for many years and eventually became a full professor at University of Toronto's medical school. He will always be remembered as a quiet, kind, and much-revered teacher. Art died at age ninety-two on June 7, 2002.

Hugh Bright, the man who revealed to me the tragic story of George and Jean Matthews, had graduated in medicine the year after Hendry. They were very good friends, and when he married in 1938, Hugh asked George to be usher at the wedding ceremony in Hart House. Hugh and his wife, Gertrude, invited Betty Summers and George to babysit their two-month-old daughter, Joanne, so they could have a little time alone together before George went off to Halifax to join the navy in late May 1941.

Hugh Bright had a long and distinguished career in senior medical administration with the RCAF in Canada and overseas. After leaving the post of commanding officer of the Institute of Aviation Medicine, he became a diplomate in health administration from the University of Toronto. As Group Captain H.J. Bright, he became the first commanding officer of the new National Defence Medical Centre in Ottawa in 1961. After retirement from the RCAF in 1967, he was medical director of Victoria Hospital in London, Ontario, for several years. Hugh Bright died in Ottawa on November 28, 1988.

After the awful news of George's death and the loneliness that followed, Betty endured another five months at Women's College Hospital doing special duty nursing in obstetrics. Finally, in March 1943, with the help of Hugh Bright (who had interceded for her with Surgeon Captain Archie MacCallum, the director of RCN Medical Services), she joined the navy's nursing service. She was posted to Halifax, to Sydney, and then back to Halifax in 1946, where she met a young RCN engineering officer, Howard Minogue. They were married in Toronto's Timothy Eaton Memorial Church on May 18, 1946. Howard took his degree in mining engineering at McGill University in 1947 and embarked on a career that took him to Washington, London, Pennsylvania, New York State, and Antarctica. He rejoined the navy in 1948 and was engineer lieutenant commander of the aircraft carrier HMCS *Magnificent* during the Korean War.

Betty had two daughters and a son: Nancy, born in 1948, Peter, in 1950, and Susie, in 1954. With Howie away overseas frequently in the 1950s, Betty purchased a house in Burks Falls, Ontario (with the money George Hendry had left her), both for her burgeoning family and for her parents. It was a happy coincidence that George's old friend and medical classmate, Hank Swan, was practising in Burk's Falls at the time; he delivered her son Peter there in 1950. Later, following Howie's very successful defence contracting business, the family moved to Washington, D.C., where Betty resumed her career as a private case room nurse for several obstetrician-gynecologists in Arlington, Virginia. In retirement there, she found a new challenge helping students, particularly international students, register for classes at Northern Virginia Community College. Finally, the family retired to Rapidan and Clark's Mountain, Virginia.

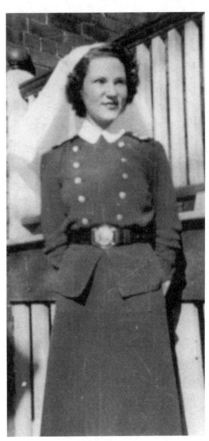

Though I talked with Betty many times by phone, I met her face to face only once, one afternoon in August 2001 in Huntsville, Ontario. She had driven down herself from Burks Falls (at age eighty-three!). We talked of George and her far too short time with him so long ago. This is a treasured memory for me.

In the fall of 2005, Betty quite suddenly developed a malignant tumour (a carcinoma) in her lung, and then, even more rapidly, an osteogenic sarcoma of her skull bone. She died at home surrounded by her family on April 10, 2006. Her daughter Susie told me, "One of the most important lessons that Mom taught me by example was to carry on and keep looking for happiness no matter what."[217] After George Hendry died, this wonderfully sweet,

Betty Summers as RCN nursing sister, 1943. (Courtesy of Betty Summers Minogue.)

gentle, and quite remarkable woman did indeed carry on, and she did find that happiness.

Carol Hendry Duffus is now the last surviving member of the Hendry family. After serving in the RCN Intelligence Branch in Halifax as a decoder (1943–1945), she met and married Alan Duffus, an architect who established a very successful firm specializing in the restoration of heritage buildings. Widowed, she lives in Waverley, Nova Scotia.

By the spring of 2001, I had determined the whereabouts of everybody even remotely connected with this story, whether alive or dead, except for Jean Matthews Hendry. The search for Jean was at once intriguing and frustrating.

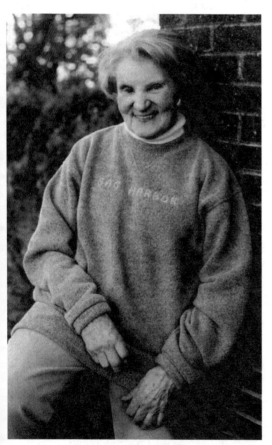

Elizabeth Audrie Summers Minogue, September 11, 1918 to April 10, 2006. (Courtesy of Susan Minogue.)

Jean had returned to Calgary at some point well before George was lost when the *Ottawa* was sunk, probably soon after a visit to Ottawa and Toronto in December 1941. Jean had moved into her mother's house at 3219 2nd Street SW in Calgary, where she was listed as living when George's death was announced in September 1942. Then, in 1945, she moved back to Vancouver with her mother. She married her second cousin, Craig Somerville,[218] on December 17, 1947, and their only child, a daughter, Margaret Gail (Maggie), was born in 1950. It was not a happy marriage and they divorced when Maggie was but seven months old. Craig Somerville died in 1964.

Sometime early in the 1970s, Jean Hendry Somerville moved into a small house in Vancouver adjoining the home of my friends Fred and Jane Bryans.[219] Jean told them both about how much she had loved George Hendry and was eager to talk about anything to do with the Toronto General Hospital. Then, in 1979, Jean moved into an apartment nearby and just dropped out of sight.

Dr. Chris Lewis, Jean's physician from 1970 till his retirement in 1985, told Jane Bryans that Jean had not been in good health and that she was probably dead. Jane and I began scouring the B.C. and Alberta Vital Statistics Agencies, B.C. Genealogy, B.C. Archives, Elections Canada, the Canadian Red Cross, and Canada411 for death statistics, addresses, and telephone numbers. This all came up empty. At this time, we had no idea of Jean's or her daughter Maggie's whereabouts.

Up one blind alley and down another. Finally, in June 2001, I talked with Chris Lewis's former secretary, Leslie Ainger. Leslie has an amazing memory and was able to confirm Jean's divorce and Craig's death, Maggie's first marriage in 1971, the birth of her two daughters and her subsequent divorce, her present marriage to a retired U.S. Navy chief petty officer (whose name, surprisingly, she couldn't remember!) in 1980, and their move to somewhere in the United States, possibly to California. Leslie recalled that Jean referred without emotion to George as "her first husband who was killed in the war." After Maggie and her family had left, Jean stayed on in Vancouver.

Then she disappeared for the second time. From all recourse we'd made to various statistical agencies and exhaustive surveys of telephone lists, we felt reasonably sure that she was not anywhere in Canada, alive or dead. The trouble was, we didn't know where to look in the U.S. Then I discovered that my cousin Ann Ward, the director of a municipal tuberculosis control agency in Toronto, and a TGH nursing graduate, was an enthusiastic and able amateur genealogist. Ann interviewed five surviving members of Jean's TGH nursing class of 1938. They agreed with the whole story, couldn't believe "that any of them could do such a thing," held George Hendry in very high regard, hadn't seen Jean in years, and thought she had probably died.

Ann's next step was to have back editions of the TGH Nursing Alumnae Association *Quarterly* searched thoroughly for news of Jean, but there was a glitch. With the demolition of the old TGH Private Patients Pavilion in April 2001, the Alumnae Association lost all their space and the entire archives with all past issues of the *Quarterly* were boxed up and stored deep in a warehouse out in Mississauga. After one false start and much further digging, Ann found a dusty copy of the February 1989 issue, which reported that Jean had died on January 4, 1989, while visiting her daughter, Maggie Frazier, who was living somewhere in California.

A U.S. search engine found Maggie's address and telephone number in Centenniel (formerly Englewood), Colorado. Maggie confirmed that her mother had been visiting her and her husband, Zane ("Zeke") Frazier, in El Toro, California, when she fell and fractured her hip. She died post-operatively on January 4, 1989. Maggie confirmed that her mother was born on June 3, 1907, and was thus eighty-one years of age when she died.

Jean had told Maggie very little about the circumstances of her marriage to George Hendry — only that she loved him very much, that she had been pregnant, and that the pregnancy had terminated in an early miscarriage. Maggie was unaware of George's engagement to Betty Summers and of George's heroism in *Ottawa*.

All very sad but perhaps not so surprising after all.

It is entirely possible that if Hugh Bright hadn't told me about that tragic encounter between George Hendry and Jean Matthews, this story would never have been told. In the event, it is rather like a play, a tragedy in two acts, linked and yet separate: one heroic and the other darker and personally devastating. One deals with the values we associate with hero-ism — a sense of duty, honour, and sacrifice. The other reveals traits like vulnerability, gullibility, ingenuousness, and a puzzling lapse of social judgement. The first is straightforward and predictable; the second is a complete enigma, a closed book.

It was tempting at first to make George Hendry the quintessential hero and cast Jean Matthews as the villain of the piece. However, for a man of his apparently sterling character and professional ability, he was surprisingly artless, and she the apparently desperate older woman, more socially advantaged than her nursing classmates and dreading the prospect of spinsterhood, who happened to stumble into an encounter that eventually ruined her and killed him.

Though he had inherited his father's wonderful capacity for friendship, George remained to the end a very private person. This was undoubtedly an act of atonement: he had to make amends for disastrously stupid mistakes. His father, W.B. Hendry, "the Chief," once wrote, "When you're wrong, admit it." George took this advice one step further and, having admitted his mistake, he was determined to make amends entirely on his own.

He felt that he'd "let the side down." He'd exposed his family's reputation to the disgrace of a scandal. He joined the navy because this would take him as far as he could possibly get from Toronto, Toronto society, the Toronto General Hospital, and his obligatory new wife. He confided in almost no one — none of his Toronto colleagues and none of his shipmates — and asked no one for help in his predicament. He offered remarkably few details of his entrapment to his mother, Betty Summers, and Hugh Bright. He may have unburdened himself to my father, his partner in practice, or to his best friend, Frank Shipp, when he visited Shipp in England just before *Ottawa's* last run. But there is little evidence of such a confidence.

He doesn't seem to have let anyone see how he felt about his mistake or about his betrayal. Henry Swan wrote to Elizabeth Hendry shortly after the news of *Ottawa's* sinking: "George never showed his feelings...." When a young colleague, Dr. Dario Carpenato, pleaded with him not to marry Jean Matthews, George told him to mind his own business.

We will never know why George was unwise enough to go alone to that party at the Toronto General in January 1941, why he didn't examine Jean to confirm or rule out a pregnancy (or have my father, his partner in practice, do so), what he told my father and what he told his best friend, Frank Shipp, when went to England shortly before the *Ottawa's* last convoy run.

I didn't begin to set the story down until many years after Hugh Bright let the genie out of the bottle. Regrettably, I let it go until much later, until many of the people who might have fleshed it out were dead. But could they have? Perhaps George didn't tell them very much after all!

After the *Ottawa* was lost, the *Toronto Daily Star* for September 21, 1942, reported that this was George's last trip "for some time," and it now seems clear that he was gong to head off on leave to Toronto to see his lawyer, W.W. McLaughlin (the same "Mr. McLaughlin" in George's letter to my father in late November 1942) and terminate "that tragic marriage," as Ralph Will had called it. He didn't hate Jean; he pitied her. He was resolutely determined to see this thing through on his own terms, to have the divorce finally settled, to get back to his practice in Toronto after the war, to be with Betty and be happy again. Out there in the dark on the North Atlantic, he was on his way back, and the most heart-rending thing about this story is that he almost made it.

Appendix A
Last Will and Testament of George Ainslie Hendry

The following will was deposited with the firm of McLaughlin, Johnston, Moorhead and Macauley, 302 Bay Street, Toronto.

THIS IS THE LAST WILL AND TESTAMENT of me, GEORGE AINSLIE HENDRY, of the City of Toronto in the County of York, Doctor of Medicine, made this 21st day of May, A.D. 1941.

1) I HEREBY REVOKE all former wills and other testamentary dispositions by me at any time heretofore made and declare this only to be and contain my Last Will and Testament.

2) I HEREBY NOMINATE, CONSTITUTE AND APPOINT my mother, ELIZABETH ROBERTSON HENDRY, and my friend, DR. JAMES C. GOODWIN to be the Executors and Trustees of this my Will, and I hereinafter refer to them as my Trustees.

3) WHEREAS I am residuary legatee under the Last Will and Testament of my aunt, JEAN A. M. McMICHAEL, I give and bequeath to my said mother, Elizabeth Robertson Hendry, the right to receive and deduct or transfer to an [...] for her own use and purposes, from the capital or corpus of the estate of my said aunt, Jean A. M. McMichael, such sum or sums without limit as to time or amount as she may decide, and I give and bequeath to her the same right in respect to my interest in the capital or corpus of the estate of my late father, William Belfry Hendry.

4) I GIVE, DEVISE AND BEQUEATH to my said Trustees, all my estate, real and personal, of every nature and kind, wheresoever situate and over which I may have power of appointment, upon the following trusts, namely:

a) TO sell, call in and convert into money all of my estate not consisting of money at such times and upon such terms as my Trustees in their discretion may decide upon with full power to postpone conversion and to retain investments in their present form as long as they deem advisable.

b) TO pay all my just debts, funeral and testamentary expenses and all succession duties and inheritance and death taxes that may be payable in connection with any insurance or any gift or benefit given by me to any person either in my lifetime or by survivorship or by this my Will or any Codicil thereto.

c) In the event of my predeceasing my mother, and subject to the later provision of this my will, to pay to <u>MISS ELIZABETH AUDREY SUMMERS</u> the sum of One Thousand Dollars ($1,000.00) and to transfer all of the remainder of my estate to my wife, <u>JEAN ISOBEL HENDRY</u>, for her sole use absolutely.

d) In the event of my mother predeceasing me to divide the remainder of my estate in the manner following:

i. One-half of the said remainder to my aunt, <u>MISS MARY DIANA HENDRY</u>, to use and dispose of as she may desire.

ii. One-quarter of the said remainder to <u>MISS ELIZABETH AUDREY SUMMERS</u>.

iii. One-quarter of the said remainder to my wife, <u>JEAN ISOBEL HENDRY</u>.

e) In the event of my predeceasing my mother and of any part of the estate of my said aunt, Jean A. M. McMichael and/or of the estate of my late father being vested in me and distributable according to my will, then I direct that that part or parts of the said estates so distributable shall be divided in the same manner namely:

i. One-half of the said remainder to my aunt, <u>MISS MARY DIANA HENDRY</u>, to use and dispose of as she may desire.

ii. One-quarter of the said remainder to <u>MISS ELIZABETH AUDREY SUMMERS</u>.

iii. One-quarter of the said remainder to my wife, <u>JEAN ISOBEL HENDRY</u>.

<u>IN WITNESS WHEREOF</u> I have hereunto set my hand this 21st day of May, A.D. 1941.

<u>SIGNED, PUBLISHED AND DECLARED</u>	)
by the said Testator as and for his Last	)
Will and Testament in the presence of us	)
both present at the same time, who, at	) George A. Hendry
his request, in his presence and in the	)
presence of each other, have hereunto	)
subscribed our names as Elizabeth	)
Robertson Hendry and James C. Goodwin.	)

Appendix B

Marriage Certificate for George Ainslie Hendry
and Jean Isobel Matthews
Preston, Ontario, April 3, 1941

REGISTERED
APR 4 1941
ON...

Jean Isobel Matthews - Nurse

I, George Ainslie Hendry, of the City of Toronto, In the Province of Ontario,
In the County of York, Surgeon, make oath and say as follows:

That, for the space of fifteen days ' immediately preceding the date of this affidavit, Jean Isobel Matthews has had her USUAL place of ABODE within the PROVINCE OF ONTARIO.

That I believe there is no kinsry, consanguinity, prior marriage or other lawful cause or legal impediment to bar or hinder the solemnization of the marriage, and

That the contents set forth herein are to the best of OUR knowledge, information and belief, true in every particular.

Names in full	George Ainslie Hendry	Jean Isobel Matthews
Occupation	Surgeon	Nurse
Age	Thirty years	Twenty-eight years
Condition	Bachelor	Spinster
Religious Denomination	United Church of Canada	Church of England in Canada.
Residence when Married	339 Walmer Rd. Toronto, Ont	Apt. 312, 219 College St. Toronto, Ontario
Place of Birth	Toronto, Ontario	Halifax, N.S.
Intended Place of Marriage	City of Toronto, County of York	In the County of York

Severally sworn before me at the City of Toronto, In the County of York, this Thirtieth day of March 1941.

_____ Deputy

_____ Issuer of Marriage License at Toronto, Ont.

Certificate of Marriage

I Certify that I solemnized the Marriage of:-

BRIDEGROOM George A. Hendry

BRIDE Jean Isobel Matthews

in the presence of

Witness _____ Preston

Address _____

Witness _____

Address _____ Preston

in the Town of Preston

County of Waterloo, PROVINCE OF ONTARIO

on the Third day of April 1941.

Name of Bridegroom's Father: William Hendry

Maiden Name of Bridegroom's Mother: _____

Name of Bride's Father: _____

Maiden Name of Bride's Mother: Jean Rebecca Bond

Address _____

Denomination: United Church of Canada

Birthplace of Bridegroom's Father	Ontario
Birthplace of Bridegroom's Mother	Ontario — Yes — Yes
Birthplace of Bride's Father	Yes

Appendix C

Letter from George Hendry to James C. Goodwin, November 23, 1941

DEPARTMENT OF NATIONAL DEFENCE
NAVAL SERVICE

Nov 23 1941
Sydney
R.C.N. Barracks

Dear Jim:-

I received your letter and one from Nels on the same day. Many thanks for the congratulations re Canadian Gynaecological Travel Society. I can see the "Goodwin touch" has again been at work. It means there's one more debt to you on my long list. Many, many thanks, though, Jim. I certainly do appreciate your kindness and thoughtfulness.

I know you're "stubborn as hell" at times. That has always been very upsetting — you're hard to convince, too — did you know?

I'll have a talk to you before long — God willing. I expect to be home on leave soon — arriving on the evening of the 15th of Dec. and leaving again a day or so after Christmas. The other party is going to Ottawa for a while and will arrive in Toronto about the 22nd. That will give me a few days at any rate. I can see Mr. McLaughlin and find out about and establish a spot of evidence before she arrives — I hope. There is a rumour to the effect that a new M.O. is coming to Sydney and that I am due to be drafted. I don't know where or when, but if I get any definite news, I'll try and leave here earlier.

It has been very pleasant here, although the work has fallen off considerably. We haven't had any surgery beyond a few toenails and infected fingers for 6 weeks.

Well, Jim, I'll be seeing you before long. Regards to Kay and the boys — also to Miss Lane and the remainder of those in the office.

As ever,
George

Appendix D
Findings of the Board of Inquiry into the Circumstances Attending the Loss of HMCS *Ottawa* on Sunday, 13 September 1942

Office of Captain (D), Newfoundland,
Old Knights of Columbus Building,
St. John's, Newfoundland
20 September 1942
cc: Flag Officer, Newfoundland Force

Sir,

We have the honour to report that we have held a full and careful investigation into the circumstances attending the loss of HMCS OTTAWA on Sunday, 13 September 1942. The Board is of the opinion that;-

HMCS OTTAWA was lost at about 2330 on 13 September 1942, due to enemy action being hit by two torpedoes at 2305 and 2320. The first torpedo striking the ship between 28 station and the stem port side. 28 bulkhead held. The second torpedo struck in the No. 2 boiler room, starboard side. The ship then listed to starboard, broke in half and sank bow and stern up. Weather — moderate sea, wind force 3, very dark, no moon.

Reconstruction of the Action.

HMCS Ottawa stationed 5000 yards ahead of convoy between 1 and 2 columns obtained two RDF contacts about green 20, 8000 yards and 6000 yards turned towards and increased to 12 and then 15 knots and set a shallow pattern. HMS WITCH, HMCS ANAPOLIS in company were expected to join convoy. WITCH had made a signal to OTTAWA "am joining and taking station 8000 yards ahead of convoy". This was inter-cepted in ST. CROIX but there is no evidence that OTTAWA received it. When RDF range had closed to about 2000 yards an object was sighted fine on the starboard bow and challenged, no reply was received. Commanding Officer appears to have been satisfied that this object was HMS WITCH as he did not order the challenge to be made again. WITCH then called up with shaded light using A's. OTTAWA replied "OTTAWA" and received "WITCH" back. The range at this time was approximately 1000 yards closing fast and OTTAWA altered to port using 20° of rudder. A/S cabinet who had reported HE on WITCH's bearing, was ordered to disregard and carry out on all round sweep for HE. After the ship had swung some 20° the first torpedo struck. Commanding Officer stopped engines, gave orders for examination and report of dam-age, prepare for abandon ship, prepare for destruction of Confidential Books and for signal "Have been torpedoed no immediate danger of sink-ing" to be passed by R/T to ST. CROIX. Depth charges were set to safe and the primers drawn by order of the First Lieutenant. It is considered that the ship continued to swing to port and lost way after turning about 180° when the U-Boat without changing position appreciably fired the second torpedo. When this torpedo had struck the ship started to list to starboard and break up. The order to abandon ship was given.

Contributing Factors.

The Commanding Officer had in mind the possibility of getting stern way on his ship but was waiting reports on damage. He appears to have expected a second torpedo. It is considered that under these circum-stances it would have been better to risk going astern in order to present a more difficult target.

Had action been sounded when RDF contacts were reported the loss of life would have been considerably less. It is estimated that approximately half the casualties were due to the explosion of the first torpedo, many of the ship's company being turned in on the mess decks at the time. The Board does not attach blame to the Commanding Officer for not sounding off action under the circumstances. The RDF contacts were obviously not a U-Boat. Two destroyers were expected from ahead and the ship's company had had little rest for some days.

Had HMCS OTTAWA been fitted with Type 271 RDF the U-Boat would probably been picked up in the sweep as well as the two destroyers.

The fact that the dark object was sighted to starboard and that an exchange of signals took place diverted most of the look out to starboard.

Signals made by WITCH were probably seen by the U-Boat and assisted in her attack.

General Remarks:

The ship was efficient and well organized as is shown by the evidence that everybody knew and carried their duties in the emergency.

The morale of the ship's company throughout was magnificent.

The Board wishes to draw special attention to the commendable devotion to duty (shown in evidence) of the following officers and men:-

The Commanding Officer, Acting Lieutenant-Commander Clark A. Rutherford, RCN and the Medical Officer, Surgeon Lieutenant George A. Hendry, RCNVR. These officers lost their lives largely through exhaustion caused by the little or no rest for some days previous. Also to Sub-Lieutenant L.B. Jenson, RCN who for a young officer displayed consider-able initiative and powers of command.

Acting Gunner (T) L.I. Jones
Petty Officer Gridel
Leading Stoker McLeod
And Sub-Lieutenant Arnold of HMS CELANDINE.

It is not clear why HMS WITCH was not aware that OTTAWA had been torpedoed.

HMS WITCH was not available at the time of the investigation.

Lessons Learned and Suggestions:

1. That the fitting of type 271 RDF to all convoy escorts and H/F-D/F FH3 to destroyers be pressed on with to the maximum.

2. That more lifesaving appliances of the float and raft types are fitted to ships and that special attention be paid to releasing launching of them. Boats in escort vessels, if not already rendered unserviceable by the stress of weather seldom get launched when the vessel is torpedoed.

3. That some secondary exit is provided in ASDIC cabinets type 124. There have been so many cases of the operators being trapped through the door becoming jammed. Ships where no deck or deckhand escape can be fitted mount removable hinge pins on the inner side so that the door can be pulled inwards if prevented by debris from opening outwards.

4. That all non-essential doors such as heads, bathroom, etc. be replaced by screens or curtains.

5. That rescue nets be made long enough to reach well below the waterline so that an exhausted man can get his feet on to something as well as his hands.

6. That the merchant service type of lifesaving jacket fitted with watertight torch be supplied to HM ships and that these jackets are fitted with a becket and toggle with which an exhausted man can secure himself to the lifesaving lanyard of a float or raft.

7. That old type of emergency rations in boats and rafts which take up a lot of space and add weight, be replaced by condensed rations.

8. That better communications to boiler rooms be fitted.

9. That in new construction, the possibility of leading pipes in living spaces along the deck instead of under the deckhead be investigated, thereby minimizing the likelihood of pinning men down when pipes fracture.

10. The merit of the old order that a sailor should always carry a knife was undoubtedly proved.

We have the honour to be,
Your obedient servants,
(Sgd) H. Frewer
Lieutenant, RCN, Member

(Sgd) R. Jackson
Lieutenant-Commander, RCNVR, Member

(Sgd) G.A. Harrison
Commander, RN, President

Appendix E
Casualty List: HMCS *Ottawa*, September 13, 1942

OFFICERS

Hendry, George Ainslie, Surgeon Lieutenant, RCNVR — Toronto, ON

McLeod, Ian S., Lieutenant, RCNVR — Haileybury, ON

Rutherford, Clark A., Lieutenant Commander, RCN — Montreal, QC

Wilson, Donald A., Sub-Lieutenant, RCN— Victoria, BC

Wright, Keith F., Sub-Lieutenant, RCNVR— Ottawa, ON

RATINGS

Adlington, Howard H., Supply Assistant — Halifax County, NS

Ashley, Robert P., Able Seaman —Winnipeg, MB

Baird, John A., Stoker — Lorneville, NB

Baker, Elgy E., Stoker — Coldwater, ON

Beddis, Samuel, Engine Room Artificer — Halifax, NS

Bell, David O., Ordinary Seaman — Toronto, ON

Bowen, Stephen D., Stoker — Toronto, ON

Bowman, Eric J., Able Seaman — Norwich, ON

Brown, Robert D., Leading Seaman — Westmount, QC

Bucheski, William, Able Seaman — Windsor, ON

Burn, Albert E., Ordinary Seaman — Vancouver, BC

Burroughs, Walter P., Able Seaman — Mitchell, ON

Campbell, Gordon K., Ordinary Seaman — Eston, SK

Campbell, Woodrow, Ordinary Seaman — Leamington, ON

Chandler, Harry M., Able Seaman — Charlottetown, PEI

Chisholm, Robert D., Able Seaman — Rineland, SK

Clemo, Frederick J. B., Able Seaman — Vancouver, BC

Collier, Chesley, Able Seaman — Halifax, NS

Collin, Joseph A. J . L., Stoker — Quebec, QC

Connolly, Richard, Leading Seaman — Halifax, NS

Coomer, Frederick, Able Seaman — Toronto, ON

Cooper, Edward B., Leading Seaman — Sudbury, ON

Cousineau, Lionel, Stoker — Lavalle County, QC

Crane, Walter J., Signalman — Hamilton, ON

Crawford, Gordon R., Petty Officer — Vancouver, BC

Creaney, Thomas, Able Seaman — Montreal, QC

Cressey, Harold F., Signalman — Toronto, ON

Cudmore, Alfred, Able Seaman — Charlottetown, PEI

Culiford, Doyle I., Stoker — Delhi, ON

Davies, William T., Able Seaman — Brandon, MB

Hunt, William E. D., Stoker — Saskatoon, SK

Deeves, Arthur J., Leading Telegraphist — Calgary, AB

Don, John R., Telegraphist — Victoria, BC

Doran, Patrick D., Stoker — Newcastle, NB

Douglas, Albert, Able Seaman — Dartmouth, NS

Dugay, Henri R., Seaman's Cook — Riviere du Loup, QC

Fisher, John A., Able Seaman — Biggar, SK

Froats, Donald McR., Officer's Cook — Belfast, Ireland

Gallagher, Howard J., Leading Seaman — Halifax, NS

Gerland, Melvin, Able Seaman — Vancouver, BC

Gibb, James A., Able Seaman — Three Rivers, QC

Glasgow, Charles E., Able Seaman — Verdun, QC

Harker, James S., Leading Telegraphist — Victoria, BC

Harris, Charles, Ordinary Seaman — Halifax, NS

Heiberg, Kenneth G., Petty Officer — Vancouver, BC

Henry, Robert, Able Seaman — Toronto, ON

Hickey, John C., Able Seaman — North Sydney, NS

Hobbis, William H., Electrical Artificer — Victoria, BC

Hockley, John W., Steward — Montreal, QC

Holmes, Earl I., Able Seaman — Swift Current, SK

Houghton, David H., Ordinary Signalman — Toronto, ON

Howard, Frederick C., Telegraphist — Winnipeg, MB

King, Arthur, Ordinary Seaman — Annapolis County, NS

Kostenki, Nicholas, Telegraphist — Clair, SK

Labonte, Ernest, Stoker — Montreal, QC

Leslie, Kenneth L., Stoker — Halifax County, NS

Leroy, Charles E., Able Seaman — Toronto, ON

Masson, Andre, Ordinary Seaman — Montreal, QC

Milburn, John R., Ordinary Artificer — Halifax, NS

Miller, Earl, Stoker — Halifax, NS

Moore, Albert A., Leading Stoker — Cowansville, QC

Morrison, Frances A., Stoker Petty Officer — Bay of Islands, NF

Morrison, Harry, Stoker — Toronto, ON

Muchmore, John V., Stoker — Victoria, BC

Murphy, Gerald W., Ordinary Seaman — Halifax, NS

MacDonald, Arthur A., Leading Supply Assistant — Mount Stewart, PEI

MacDonald, Hubert, C., Chief Stoker — Victoria, BC

MacKenzie, Charles A., Leading Seaman — Long Branch, ON

McKechnie, Morton H., Ordinary Seaman — Regina, SK

MacMillan, Alexander, Sick Berth Attendant — Kingston, ON

Neath, John F. E., Able Seaman — Owen Sound, ON

Neil, Percy T., Able Seaman — Woodroofe, ON

Palmer, Ralph B. N., Able Seaman — Winnipeg, MB

Paradis, Paul V., Able Seaman — Montreal, QC

Peppler, Stanley, Able Seaman — Listowell, ON

Pettitt, John B., Stoker — Kingston, ON

Piontek, Jack W., Able Seaman — Toronto, ON

Pooles, Donald H., Telegraphist — Winnipeg, MB

Porter, Harold S., Ordinary Seaman — Toronto, ON

Purcell, Herbert A., Engine Room Artificer — Halifax, NS

Quigley, Lloyd P. W., Able Seaman — Vancouver, BC

Rasmussen, Clifford J., Ordinary Seaman — St. James, MB

Riches, Clifford, Able Seaman — Toronto, ON

Robertson, Earl J., Coder — Winnipeg, MB

Robinson, Walter V. D., Able Seaman — Victoria, BC

Robshaw, George A., Able Seaman — Montreal, QC

Roop, Roy M., Able Seaman — Annapolis County, NS

Secord, Gerard F., Able Seaman — Saint John, NB

Sheppard, David G., Leading Signalman — Winnipeg, MB

Shillito, John G., Able Seaman — Union Bay, BC

Simons, Clinton L,. Ordinary Signalman — Swift Current, SK

Slaunwhite, Harry M., Able Seaman — Halifax, NS

Smith, Alexander, Able Seaman… — Winnipeg, MB

Smith, Arthur, Able Seaman — Brandon, MB

Smith, Kenneth G., Seaman's Cook — New Westminster, BC

Smith, Roseville St. Clair, Stoker — Athleston, QC

Southall, Harry K., Able Seaman — Halifax, NS

Stephens, Oswald B., Stoker — Long Beach, ON

Taylor, Ernest F., Able Seaman — Livingstone, Louisiana, USA

Taylor, Frederick F. M., Ordinary Seaman — Essex, ON

Trainor, Alfred N., Petty Officer Steward — Armdale P.O., NS

Tremblay, Joseph A. S., Able Seaman — Charlevoix County, QC

Trudel, Camille G., Stoker — Quebec, QC

Whiting, Basil E., Able Seaman — Whaletown, BC

Wilson, Archibald W., Stoker — Victoria, BC

Young, Thomas W., Able Seaman — Hamilton, ON

Zinck, Cyril M., Supply Assistant — Halifax, NS

Died of wounds received in action:

Emerslund, Arnold G., Telegraphist — Vancouver, BC

Appendix F
List of Survivors: HMCS *Ottawa*, September 13, 1942

OFFICERS

Sub-Lieutenant Thomas Hugh Buchanan, RCNVR
Sub-Lieutenant Latham Brereton Jenson, RCN
Lieutenant Joseph A.J.D. Lantier, RCN
Lieutenant (E) Donald Lachlan McGillivray, RCNVR
Lieutenant Thomas Charles Pullen, RCN

RATINGS

Abwheeler, Vernon, Engine Room Artificer, 3rd Class, V-22137, RCNVR
Acton, Robert G., Able Seaman, V-18199, RCNVR
Archibald, Herbert L., Able Seaman, 3124, RCN
Barriault, Michael, Acting Leading Steward, A-2961, RCNR
Billard, Robert A., Shipwright 3rd Class, 40663, RCN
Carracher, F., Cook, V-1521, RCNVR
Causley, John L., Supply Assistant, V-19414, RCNVR
Currie, Patrick D., Petty Officer, 2800, RCN
Doucette, Wilfred U., Able Seaman, A-4762, RCNR
Dobing, Sydney R., Able Seaman, 4729, RCN
Eagle, Frederick W., Chief Engine Room Artificer, 21549, RCN
Fraser, Alexander, Ordinary Seaman, V-326, RCNVR
Fox, Edward R., Able Seaman, V-22894, RCNVR
Gignac, Robert H., Stoker, V-19217, RCNVR
Grivel, George Q., Petty Officer, 2534, RCN
Hard, Arthur A., Acting Petty Officer, 3267, RCN
Hawkins, George H., Stoker, V-18463, RCNVR
Hood, Patrick A., Leading Seaman, 2486, RCN
Hunter, Herbert, Ordinary Seaman, V-14625, RCNVR
Jones, Lloyd Irwin, Gunner (T), RCN
Johnson, George D., Stoker, V-8887, RCNVR
Joseph, Aurelle F., Able Seaman, 4248, RCN
Kirkpatrick, James J., Steward, V-13662, RCNVR

Leighton, Thomas A., Signalman, V24029, RCNVR

Locke, Maurice M., Engine Room Artificer 3rd Class, 21650, RCN

Logos, Steve, Ordinary Seaman, 4349, RCN

MacKinnon, Duncan L., Ordinary Seaman, V-10550, RCNVR

Mason, Roy A., Leanding Cook (S), A-834, RCNR

McCauley, Henry A., Able Seaman, V-6239, RCNVR

McGiven, George H., Leading Stoker, 21592, RCN

McLaurin, Donald, Writer, V-6440, RCNVR

McLeod, Malcolm A., Leading Stoker, 21759, RCN

McQueen, William S., Leading Signalman, V-2110, RCNVR

Owen, Mervyn, Able Seaman, 4252, RCN

Paradis, Anthony G., Supply Assistant, 40719, RCN

Patten, Kenneth, Cook (O), V-13806, RCNVR

Parent, Joseph N., Stoker 2nd Class, V-3723, RCNVR

Reeves, Douglas H., Able Seaman, 4254, RCN

Rollinson, Frederick M., Able Seaman, 2581, RCN

Seath, Ritchie O., Coder, V-23611, RCNVR

Scott, Peter W., Able Seaman, V-7623, RCNVR

Sinclair, Roy C., Acting Stoker Petty Officer, 21564, RCN

Skillen, Clement R., Able Seaman, V-16231, RCNVR

Smith, Cecil, Acting Engine Room Artificer 3rd Class, V-30468, RCNVR

Smith, John, Petty Officer, 1861, RCN

Soles, Norman S., Able Seaman, 3811, RCN

Stone, Douglas B., Able Seaman, 4222, RCN

Taylor, David S., Petty Officer, 3393, RCN

Terrabassi, Joseph, Ordinary Seaman, V-19351, RCNVR

Thomas, Fernand, Ordinary Seaman, 4171, RCN

Thomas, Richard H., Acting Stoker Petty Officer, V15131, RCNVR

Tizzard, John, Acting Stoker Petty Officer, 21456, RCN

Underhill, Alvin R., Able Seaman, 4268, RCN

Waller, James, Acting Petty Officer Cook (S), 40507, RCN

Waycik, Walter E., Able Seaman, V-22866, RCNVR

Wedmark, Alvin G., Able Seaman, V-9592, RCNVR

Weir, Robert R., Able Seaman, V-17167, RCNVR

Williamson, John N., Stoker, V-1680, RCNVR

Wilson, John E., Stoker, V-12367, RCNVR

Wilson, Norman, Able Seaman, V-14397, RCNVR

Withus, Alfred S., Able Seaman, V16464, RCNVR

Works, Harlan, Stoker, V-26154, RCNVR

Worth, Elton, Able Seaman, V-1227, RCNVR

Wortman, George E., Acting Stoker Petty Officer, 21200, RCN

Walterson, Gudmund J., Acting Leading Stoker, V-2201, RCNVR

Appendix G

Report of Proceedings for Task Unit 24.1.14 Escorting Convoy ON 127:
HMCS *St. Croix* (LCdr. A.H. Dobson, DSC, RCNR,
Commanding Officer)

17 September, 1942

FROM: The Commanding Officer
HMCS "ST. CROIX"

TO: The Captain (D) Newfoundland
Old Knights of Columbus Bldg.
St. John's, Newfoundland

COPY: The Director of Anti-Submarine Warfare
Admiralty, Bath, England

REPORT OF PROCEEDINGS — TASK UNIT 24.1.14

ESCORTING CONVOY ON 127

---

1. Task unit 24.1.14, consisting of HMC Destroyers "St. Croix" and "Ottawa" and Corvettes "Sherbrooke", "Arvida", "Amherst" and HMS "Celandine" sailed from Loch Foyle, Northern Ireland at 0730B the 5th September.

2. Clyde section of convoy was sighted at 1035B and at 1135B Task unit joined main section of convoy. Convoy papers were received from HMS "Mold". At 1845 Loch Ewe section joined and course was altered to 262° with escorts in NE 6 & DE 6, WACI's.

At 1435Z the 10th, when in DE 6, three ships, pennants 12, 22, & 32 were torpedoed. #12 was torpedoed on the starboard side whereas

#22 & #32 were torpedoed on the port side. This indicated that 2 submarines were attacking. Sherbrooke was ordered to stand by ships torpedoed; St. Croix, Celandine and Ottawa turned towards convoy and carried out sweep. At 1525Z St. Croix fired a medium patter on a contact. #22 was able to continue in convoy but pennants 12 and 32 appeared to be hopeless. Sherbrooke was ordered to sink the freighter. Ottawa ordered to take up station at visibility distance astern in order to prevent submarine surfacing and following convoy.

3. At 1656Z Arvida attacked a good contact with a 10 charge pattern. 1913Z, St. Croix who had been gathering information from port wing ships as to previous attack, had A/S contact at 1000 yards ahead of Commodore but was unable to turn quickly enough so passed down between columns 5 & 6. At 1915 EMPIRE OIL was torpedoed on starboard quarter and about 4 minutes later was torpedoed on port bow. The contact St. Croix had was classified as doubtful but it was evidently a submarine which passed down between #4 & #5 columns of convoy. The periscope of a submarine was observed in the convoy close to the Empire Oil after it was torpedoed and St. Croix turned and went up between #4 & #5 columns obtaining an echo range 800 yards at 1918Z. St. Croix fired a shallow pattern and regained contact distant 600 yards bearing 140° on which a medium pattern was fired. Celandine and St. Croix carried out search astern of convoy and Ottawa, who had come up by this time carried out an attack on a contact. Celandine was ordered to rejoin convoy but got a contact and searched until about 2151Z when ordered to return to convoy to take charge.

4. Ottawa screened St. Croix when picking up survivors from Empire Oil and herself picked up 1 boat load, being screened by St. Croix. At 2130Z St. Croix and Ottawa proceeded to rejoin convoy.

5. At 2225Z star shells and snow flakes were observed ahead and signals received from Celandine saying that a ship had been torpedoed. This was #84. At 2345 star shells were again observed and evidently, about this time, #23 was torpedoed. At 2355 an RDF contact obtained bearing 140At 2225Z star shells and snow flakes were observed ahead and

signals received from Celandine saying that a ship had been torpedoed. This was #84. At 2345 star shells were again observed and evidently, about this time, #23 was torpedoed. At 2355 an RDF contact obtained bearing 140° at 1 ? miles. Course was altered towards, target was closed at 2359 wake of a submarine was observed close on the starboard beam proceeding in the opposite direction. A shallow pattern was fired but no contact was regained. Course was then set to rejoin convoy.

6. At 0125Z the 11th, Arvida reported sighting a submarine on the surface 1000 yards and attacked with a 10 charge pattern believed successful. About this time Amherst also attacked contact on Port bow. At 0145Z Ottawa attacked contact on Port quarter but was not promising and contact was not regained.

7. At 0200Z Sherbrooke who had been sinking torpedoed ships reported she was 25 miles astern of convoy and rejoining. She was then ordered to stand by any torpedoed ships which she saw on her way back to convoy. The remaining escorts were put in position NE 5.

8. At 0321 Celandine attacked a submarine on the surface with very promising results.

9. Escort diagram DE 5, WACI's was used the next day as Sherbrooke had not yet rejoined. Pennants 84 which had been torpedoed the previous night was still slightly astern of the convoy and regained station.

10. At 1450Z the 11th Ottawa attacked a doubtful contact ahead of columns 3 & 4. At 1600 St. Croix proceeded to visibility distance ahead of convoy in order to scout. At 1716 ability distance ahead of convoy in order to scout. At 1716 a submarine was sighted on the surface bearing 340°. Altered course toward and chased it at full speed. At 1755Z #11 was torpedoed on starboard side. At 1749 submarine which was being chased, dived. St. Croix searched area but failed to regain contact. At this time a suspicious merchant vessel was in sight and signal was made reporting it.

11. At 1928 Amherst was ordered to sink #11 and return to the convoy. At 2135Z, St. Croix when returning to convoy investigated an RDF contact without results. At 2235Z convoy was attacked and 2 ships torpedoed. At this time St. Croix and Amherst were away from convoy. Arvida was ordered to stand by torpedoed ships. At 0034Z the 12th Emperor Thackery Pennants 24 reported hitting a submerged object, impact not severe, object scraped along the bottom for about 30 feet.

12. At 0100 the 12th St. Croix rejoined convoy. At 0127 pennants #42 was torpedoed and was reported by Arvida to be listing heavily and that she had picked up survivors. #31, the other ship torpedoed was reported with engine room flooded and not likely to sink and also that confidential books were still on board. This ship was later reported on fire and sinking.

13. At 0139Z Sherbrooke reported dropping 2 charges on a contact. At 0238Z, Arvida reported attacking a submarine on the surface. At 0417Z convoy was again attacked and #64 was torpedoed. Operation Raspberry was carried out without success.

15. [sic]   At 0630Z the 12th, Arvida who had been standing by the torpedoed ships, reported having made 2 promising attacks; one in which a U-boat at 1000 yards ahead of Celandine, following convoy at 14 knots, crash dived when range 500 yards, made a good attack with shallow pattern which blew it to the surface. It submerged again at 600 yards and a good attack was carried out after which contact disappeared. At 0445Z Celandine sighted another submarine on the surface and attacked. Submarine crash dived and Celandine attacked with depth charges. At 0712 Celandine was ordered to rejoin convoy.

16. At 0835 escorts were ordered to take station ahead of convoy, destroyers on each wing and 2 corvettes in the centre as it was felt that all daylight attacks had come from ahead.

That morning Arvida reported that when standing by burning EMPIRE MOONBEAM she had sighted a submarine on the surface at 1000 yards, submarine crash dived and Arvida carried out a good attach with a 6 charge pattern, two heavy underwater explosions were heard after charges exploded. Contact was not regained.

17. At 1318Z when stationed 2000 yards ahead of #3 column Arvida reported she believed she had contact with a submarine and made an attack. At 1418Z Celandine reported sighting a submarine astern of the convoy and St. Croix sighted one bearing 280°. Again at 1537Z sighted one bearing 010°. At 1748Z a submarine was observed bearing 290° seven miles from convoy. At 1750Z St. Croix increased [to] 20 knots and at 1755 submarine dived. At 1800Z St. Croix resumed zig-zag on starboard bow of convoy.

18. At 1849Z submarine echo bearing 190° was gained and at 1857Z pattern set to 50 feet was fired on this contact. St. Croix then turned round and passed down between columns 5 & 6 of convoy. At 1905Z contact was gained but it was decided this was not a sub and was not attacked. At this time Celandine who was astern of #6 column reported HE [hydrophone effect] and there is no doubt felt that this was the submarine which had attempted attack on the convoy.

19. At 0455Z/13 RDF contact bearing 270°, 3 miles was investigated and found to be the Ottawa. No attacks were made on the convoy during the night nor during the following day.

20. At 2314Z/13 HMS "Witch" reported she was 10,000 yards ahead of convoy and "Annapolis" 2 miles on port beam. At 2325 St. Croix signalled Witch "Propose you take position A, NE 8; Annopolis C". Witch agreed and signalled "Please remain senior officer until morning."

21. At 2352Z Ottawa reported investigating 2 suspicious RDF contacts 5 miles ahead of convoy. It was presumed that these were Witch and Annapolis and signal was made to that effect.

22. At 0005Z/14 Witch reported by RT "Believe Ottawa torpedoed". Shortly after this 2 white rockets were observed ahead and St. Croix

increased to 15 knots and sighted Ottawa on port bow within 4 or 5 minutes. She was on an even keel and appeared not badly damaged. St. Croix swept up towards Ottawa on her starboard side and had reached a position on her starboard bow when an explosion believed to be from a torpedo, took place at 0016. St. Croix then passed ahead of Ottawa and when sweeping her port side, observed her to sink. Signal was made to Celandine ordering her to close at best speed and to Commodore ordering emergency turn to starboard. Flares were observed in the water where Ottawa had sunk.

23. At 0034Z/14th St. Croix picked up HE bearing 210° and proceeded to investigate ordering Celandine to search for survivors, Arvida to screen her whilst doing so. At 0035 echo bearing 180° very slight was obtained. [*sic*] At 0041 echo was lost but fast HE was heard. It appeared the submarine was at periscope depth as no RDF contact could be gained. Speed was increased to 15 knots, occasionally reducing to 10 knots in order to verify HE bearing. At 0055 an echo was gained bearing 210°, 1100 yards. At 0058Z ? a medium pattern was fired.

24. At 0105Z Arvida reported "Tanker torpedoed on starboard side survivors in water and in boats, proceeding to Ottawa". At 0110Z RDF contact was gained near where charges had been dropped and fast HE heard. St. Croix increased to full speed and gradually closed target until finally at 0115, wake and conning tower of submarine was sighted close under port bow. A round was fired from #3 gun and a star shell fired from #1 gun but it was not felt that this was effective as the gun's crew could not see the target. The submarine crash dived when about 20 yards ahead of the bow and a pattern set to 100 feet was fired at 0117Z. No further contact was gained.

25. At 0135Z, St. Croix stopped engines when in vicinity of flares, men were observed in the water and on rafts. St. Croix ordered Arvida "Close me near torpedoed tanker so as to screen me whilst we pick up survivors". At 0140Z St. Croix proceeded ahead to clear rafts as it was thought too dangerous to remain stopped when submarines were in

the vicinity. At this time it was thought that the survivors were from the torpedoed tanker which was fairly close but since then it appears that they were from the Ottawa.

26. At 0157Z an echo bearing 220° 1100 yards was gained but was very shortly lost. At 0221Z, commenced screening Celandine and Arvida who were picking up survivors. At 0240Z echo bearing 270° 1200 yards was gained. At 0242Z ? echo was bearing 250° distance 300 yards. Contact was lost at 200 yards and at 0243 ? medium pattern fired. At 0247Z contact was regained 050° distance 900 yards but was quickly lost.

27. At 0301Z Arvida reported she was screening Celandine. At 0327Z St. Croix ordered Celandine and Arvida to pick up survivors and signalled that we were screening. At 0336Z Annapolis, who was in vicinity was ordered to return to convoy.

28. At 0404Z an echo was gained range 1100 yards, closed contact and prepared to attack. At 0405Z echo was bearing 018° range 500 yards, 0405Z ? range 300 yards lost contact, 0407Z fired deep pattern of 4 charges. 4 charges only were used as this would leave St. Croix with 2 charges for any further attacks. These charges exploded and a fifth explosion was heard which did not appear to be the usual depth charge explosion. Contact was regained on charges and whilst following in, another contact was obtained beyond the charges. At 0415Z echo bearing 177° range 1300 yards was obtained but was lost at 0416Z range 1000 yards the echo gradually fading away. St. Croix searched the area then returned to screen Celandine and Arvida.

29. At 0755Z the 14th, daylight, St. Croix prepared to put Doctor on board Arvida, this operation was completed at 1035Z when Celandine and Arvida left at best speed for St. John's. St. Croix searched area until 1300Z without sighting further survivors when course was set for St. John's.

30. St. Croix secured alongside Harvey's #3 wharf to land survivors at 1556Z the 15th. Distance travelled 2811.7 miles, fuel remaining 3 tons, Depth charges remain — 2.

31. Daylight attacks appeared to come from submarines which came into the convoy from ahead and it is considered that the screen is in WACI's leaves the front exposed to this form of attack. There being only 3 ships to screen an area about 5 miles in extent. In some of the night attacks, it appeared that the submarines had come in from ahead of the convoy but there seems no doubt that the submarines remained in the vicinity of torpedoed ships for some time and overtook the convoy by coming up astern.

32. When at least 4 escorts were ahead of the convoy and the convoy had been reduced to a front of 3 to 4 miles, it is considered that 2 attacks by submarines were prevented as Arvida attacked a submarine close ahead of the convoy in the morning and St. Croix attached a definite submarine, close ahead of the convoy in the afternoon. Amherst also reported attacking a contact in the same position shortly after.

33. It is considered that St. Croix, Celandine and Arvida all made very good attacks with a good possibility of success.

(Sgd.) A.H. Dobson
Lieut. Commander, RCNR

Appendix H

Report of Proceedings: HMS *Witch*,
C 4 Escort Group for Convoy ON 127
(LCdr. S.R.J. Woods, RNR, Commanding Officer)

CONVOY ON 127

HMS "WITCH"

18th September 1942

Sir,

I have the honour to forward the following report of proceedings of HMS "WITCH", under my command, for the period from 2200Z on Saturday September 12th, to 1830Z on Friday September 19th.

2. Saturday September 12th. 2200Z Task Unit 24.18.2, consisting HMS "WITCH" (Senior Officer) and HMC Ships "ANNAPOLIS", "MONCTON", REGINA", and "BRANTFORD" sailed from St. John's, NF. On clearing harbour, "WITCH" and "ANNAPOLIS" proceeded at 17? knots to reinforce escort with Convoy, as it was being attacked, corvettes proceeding under their own Senior Officer in "MONCTON".

3. Sunday September 13th. 0900Z. Increased to 19.4 knots in order to join Convoy before dark, but owing to Convoy being late, junction was not effected until 2250Z, in position 47 degrees 54 minutes North, 42 degrees 15 minutes West.

4. Monday September 14th. 0000Z. Contacted HMCS "OTTAWA" who had come ahead of convoy to investigate suspicious contact, which was believed to be "WITCH".

0003Z. With "WITCH" in position approximately 270 degrees 10,000 yards from leading ship of starboard wing column, "OTTAWA" was silhouetted by a large explosion, which appeared to take place in vicinity of port side of her after funnel. "WITCH", assuming "OTTAWA" to be torpedoed, fired two white rockets, informed HMCS "ST. CROIX" (CTU 24.1.14) by R/T that "OTTAWA" was believed to be torpedoed. Course was immediately altered and a sweep carried out across head of Convoy to the port bow, back to vicinity of "OTTAWA", and down starboard side of Convoy. (See track chart).

0300Z. "WITCH" took station 3 miles ahead of Convoy, which at this time was being escorted by HMCS "AMHERST" and "SHER-BROOKE". Remainder of escorts had appeared to concentrate to the south-eastward, where starshell, gunflashes, and searchlights were observed. During this period reports were being received from other escorts that a tanker had also been torpedoed. These were afterwards found to be incorrect, but were caused by the tanker "CLAUSINA" stopping to pick up "OTTAWA"'s survivors, but, on seeing corvettes, regained her station on Convoy. Weather during this period:- Wind, South-west, force 4-5, sea moderate, short moderate swell, very dark but clear.

1320Z. "ANNAPOLIS", who was running short of fuel, due to continuous steaming at high speed, was detached to St. John's, NF to fuel. Escort throughout remainder of day consisted of "WITCH", "AMHERST" and "SHERBROOKE".

5. Friday September 18th. 0250Z. White light was observed bearing 340 degrees. "ANNAPOLIS" ordered to investigate. This was found to be a Portuguese fishing vessel.

6. 1000Z. Relief escort consisting of HM Ships "MONTGOMERY" and "ROXBURGH" and HMC Ships "BILLE DE QUEBEC" and "SHEDIAC" joined and took over, in position 43 degrees 23 minutes North, 61 degrees 42 minutes West.

1010Z. HMS "WITCH", who was running short of fuel proceeded to Halifax with SS "BAYANO", leaving "ANNAPOLIS" and remainder of group to escort Halifax portion of Convoy, consisting of 4 ships.

1830Z. Arrived at Halifax NS.

7. <u>REMARKS.</u>

(i) Considering the trying period through which Convoy had passed, it was considered that discipline and station-keeping was excellent.

(ii) SS "CLAUSINA"'s conduct on the early morning of 14th September, in stopping to attempt the rescue of survivors from "OTTAWA", despite the believed presence of U-boats, is considered worthy of mention.

(iii) Attached is the list of ships torpedoed and missing. This information was obtained from Commodore.

(iv) With reference to Captain (D) Halifax's D.13-1-3 of 14th April 1942, no excessive traffic was intercepted on 2410 kcs.

I have the honour to be, Sir,
Your obedient Servant,

(Signed) S. R. J. WOODS
Lieutenant Commander RNR

The Commanding Officer, Atlantic Coast
HMC Dockyard
Halifax, NS

Appendix I

Excerpts from U-91's *Kriegstagebuch* (War Diary)
(Oblt. z. S. Heinz Walkerling, Commanding Officer)
and *Schussmeldung für*
Überwasserstreitkräfte und U-boote, 14.9.42
(Shot Report for Surface Forces and Submarines)

U-91 had sailed from Kiel on 15 August 1942 for her first patrol. She joined the Vorwärts Group in a long patrol line West of Ireland on 27 August. Another boat on line sighted convoy SC 97 on 31 August and Walkerling and others closed. He sighted the convoy later the same day at 1720 but was driven off by an escort. The next day he was forced down by aircraft four times. He regained contact with the convoy at 2105 but was then surprised [the KTB honestly says just that] by an aircraft coming out of a low cloud bank. The aircraft dropped 3 bombs which exploded when U-91 was down to 60 m, causing minor damage. Walkerling again lost contact for 3 hours but sighted "destroyers" at 0040 on the 2nd and then the convoy itself at 0700. He promptly attacked at 0715, firing a salvo of 4 torpedoes but all missed [presumably because they had been fired from 3,000 metres]. It was now too light for a surface attack and U-91 dived. Shortly afterwards BdU ordered boats not well placed for submerged attacks to break off to the West.

On 2 September the KTB records a message from BdU ordering 13 boats into a new Vorwärts patrol line. U-91 was to be the 5th boat in from the Northern end of the line. The patrol line was told that a westbound convoy was expected to pass through its area on the 4th.

On the 4th BdU ordered the line to shift to the SW at 6 knots for 11? hours commencing at 2200. Boats were to start patrolling their new stations at 0930 on the 5th.

The KTB records the same reports that a convoy had been sighted by boats at the southern end of the line found in U-218's KTB. Oblt.

Walkerling stated moving SW at 1118 on the 6th. He was in thick fog but the KTB does not include sea state or wind force. These were apparently more benign than those being encountered by U-218 further to the N.

At 1129 on the 7th boats were told to break off and to resume their old sequence on a line from AK 5664 to AL 7854.

On 9 September U-584 (Deecke) at the southern end of the line reported sighting ON 127 at 2100.

By 1600 on the 10th Walkerling calculated that he was 30 nm SW of the convoy. He apparently sighted it at 1907:

10.9.42

1907	Transmitted message in short code: Have contact with convoy in Qu AK 9945.
2000	AK 9861
2219	Received radio message 2224 To Mumm, Walkerling, Ölrich. Transmit shadowing reports immediately. If reports not heard other boats are to transmit.
	I therefore sent the following:
2334	Signal in short code: In contact, Qu 9885, course 200.
2400	With the onset of darkness I close in to attack.

11.9.42

At 0430 U-91 reported that she had been driven off by an escort, but at

0800 the KTB records regaining contact at morning twilight. Oblt. Walkerling then sent shadowing reports at 2 hour intervals.

U-91 dived for a submerged attack at 2050 when the convoy made an alteration of course to the south. She closed in to 8,000 m and observed a twin-funnelled destroyer of the "D class" ahead and a four-funnelled destroyer stationed close on his side with an escort stationed further out [presumably Ottawa and St. Croix]. Walkerling counted approximately 20 merchant ships including 2 large tankers. However, when Walkerling took an all-round look he noticed an escort from 500 m on his starboard beam and closing. The CO went to 50 m and listened. When the bearing of the escort drew forward he returned to periscope depth to find that he was no longer favourably placed.

U-91 surfaced at 2356 and reported having been driven off during an attempted attack during daylight.

12.9.42

At 0400 on the 12th the KTB records that U-91 had penetrated through the screen for a night attack. Escorts were seen on the port bow and starboard quarter. However, illumination rockets were fired by the convoy and the boat was apparently spotted by an escort. Walkerling turning away at ? speed but the escort followed and opened fire with a gun at a range of 600 m. The escort stationed on the bow now fired starshells.

U-91 carried out an emergency dive at 0513 and went to 140 m. 11 depth charges exploded, causing slight damage.

Escorts using ASDIC were heard and at 0715 5 more depth charges exploded. U-91 surfaced at 0930 when the last ship noises faded and reported the attack at 1138. The insulation around 36 battery cells had been cracked.

At 1137 on the 13th a "destroyer" which closed rapidly was sighted. Walkerling dived at 1207 but no depth charges followed. She was back on the surface at 1440 and again pursued. Oblt. Walkerling sighted the convoy itself at 2352 just as it was making an alteration of course, but lost contact again. However at 0150 on the 14th he again sighted silhouettes and attacked.

14.9.42

0150 (This was European central time which was 3 hours beyond the local time, therefore the local time was 2250.)

I sight several silhouettes and must be positioned directly ahead of the convoy. I discern a twin-funnelled destroyer at slow speed far ahead of the convoy on inclination 70. Fired salvo of two torpedoes at the destroyer from Tubes I and III. Target speed — 11 knots, range — 1000 m, inclination — red 70, lead angle — 4 degrees, depth — 2 m.

0215 Two explosions after 1 minute 50 seconds. Black and white explosive cloud and bright red flames. The destroyer lies stopped burning heavily and fires a shell which splits into 5 green stars. Starshells are immediately fired from other vessels. I assume that this is an emergency signal as a second destroyer proceeds to the position from which it was fired. I turn a full circle using maximum helm and commence a new approach towards the second destroyer which is now lying stopped. Fired a single shot from Tube II with firing angle 0 degrees. Running time 1 minute 45 seconds, hit amidships. Tall water column. Several explosions in succession. These appear to be exploding depth charges. The destroyer sank immediately. Considerable fireworks, starshells. On completion of a

242

five-starred rocket, the position from which it was fired is swept by a search light. 3 to 4 escorts simultaneously switch on green-red lights at the mastheads and fire red stars. After roughly 2 minutes, the lights are switched off. I am still located inside the defences and proceed towards the dark horizon at ½ speed. I again penetrate into the convoy but am driven off by the firing of starshells and searching with search lights. A maximum helm and lose the destroyer from sight.

I observe an additional torpedo hit from another boat on a merchant ship.

The convoy has dropped back markedly with respect to me and I lose contact. I pursue on a westerly course.

0400 — BC 6148

0800 Qu 5329 — SSW 4, 10/10 overcast, seastate 3-4, rain showers, visibility rapidly deteriorating.

0630 — Transmitted Radio Message 0602:
Hit twin-funnelled destroyer with salvo of two torpedoes, target burning heavily, hit second destroyer which went alongside amidships. This target sank immediately. Sinking of the first destroyer not observed because of increasing threat from escorts. SSW 3, 15 mb (millibars, for pressure), heavy rain, 5+ torpedoes, 28 cu. m, continuing to operate against convoy.

1125 — Received Radio Message 1029:
1. Continue the pursuit, remain tough.
2. Replenishment will occur in BC 9355. Break off so that replenishment location can be reached with minimum reserve of fuel.

3; On breaking off operation each boat is to report fuel and torpedo states and readiness for action.

(Heavy fog was encountered commencing at 1200 along with heavy rain. U-91 broke off the operation at 2048, refuelled from U-461 NW of the Azores and reached Brest on 6 October.)

Remarks by Flag Officer Submarines Concerning KTB for "U-91" for the periods 15.8–7.10.1942:

1.) This was the first patrol by this Commanding Officer with a new boat.

2.) The operations against convoys were affected by bad weather and poor visibility conditions.

3.) The boat permitted herself to be frequently surprised by surface and air forces.

4.) The Commanding Officer exploited the opportunity for success on 14.9 fully and achieved the very gratifying success of sinking two destroyers.

5.) The experiences gained during this patrol against convoys will be considerable value during future patrols.

Seen in draft by: D ö n i t z
Certified correct: (Signature) Lt. And Adjutant

Appendix J

Transcript of a Taped Interview of
Captain T.C. Pullen, OC, RCN (Ret'd)
by Commander Tony German, RCN (Ret'd), on January 26, 1985

GERMAN: Tom, could you tell us the story, as you saw it, of the action around Convoy ON127, 13th September, 1942?

PULLEN: Convoy ON127 [that indicated a westbound convoy, mostly with empty ships] was a largish convoy and was subjected to a U-Boat attack in mid-Atlantic, an attack that went on for 5 or 6 days, and all together, we had been shadowed, and then attacked by a total of 13 U-Boats. This was the first experience I had had in a ship and in a convoy subject to attack, and in the OTTAWA we were ahead of the convoy on the night of September 13, and looking for supporting ships coming out to meet us from St. Johns, Newfoundland. It was in that position, ahead of the convoy about 11:20 at night, we were hit by a torpedo.

GERMAN: Could you perhaps give us some events that preceded that?

PULLEN: Yes it was, it was quite an interesting period, because shortly after we had sailed from Londonderry on the 5th of September, and we were several days at sea, one of our men came down with acute appendicitis and the doctor on board, Surgeon Lt. GEORGE HENDRY, an outstanding man, decided that if we couldn't go back, he would have to operate, and he did, and I volunteered to assist, and it was carried out on the table in the Captain's cabin, and went on for 3 hours, and was entirely successful, and a great education for me. After that, with the first attack on the convoy took place

245

on the 9th of September and on the 10th, a ship called the EMPIRE OIL was torpedoed and we picked up some of her survivors, one of whom had a very serious injury, a rivet had been blown into his gut, and the next day the doctor said it was a very serious situation and he would have to operate to remove the rivet and would I act as assistant again. I seem to be proof against the whole horrible business, and he operated on this man for 4 hours, but unfortunately it was not successfully and on Sunday on the 13th in the morning he died of peritonitis and we buried him that night at sunset on the quarterdeck on the ship, and at 5 minutes past 11, the men who were standing on the quarterdeck a few hours before were themselves blown up at 5 past 11.

GERMAN: Were you just completely alone when you were torpedoed? You had no prior warning or anything?

PULLEN: No, we had left our station in front of the convoy and gone ahead about 10 or 15 miles, to seek a rendezvous with a destroyer coming — the destroyer WITCH coming out from St. Johns, and of course in those days the U-Boats gathered ahead of the convoy in preparation for the night attack, and of course what we did was blunder into the marshalling area, I suppose you could call it, and U-91 detected us and fired 2 torpedoes, one of which hit the bow of the ship, blew the front end of the ship right off, and at the time I was standing on the quarterdeck, because I was expecting something to happen, I had heard the ships propellers increase speed, and that's always a sign to people sleeping below that something is in the wind, and it was while I was standing there that first explosion shattered the night, and shattered me.

GERMAN: And how quickly did the ship go down?

PULLEN: Well of course this didn't inflict a fatal wound to the ship. We still had our propulsion system, but we were dead in the water and I went up onto the bridge and reported to the Captain, LARRY RUTHERFORD, and it had been a long and grim time for him, this attack had been going on for days, and he was very tired, but I went down below to inspect the damage and to make a report to him, and we lay wallowing in the sea while (there was one other person, and I can't remember who it is now) we went down into what was left of the forward lower Messdecks, and it was a scene of carnage and shambles, and we were scrambling around there in the wreckage and you could see the sea just straight ahead of the ship, where the bow used to be, and I had that awful feeling that if there was one torpedo, there could be another, and why wasn't the ship moving, going astern to get out of the way and present a moving target, and when the 2nd torpedo hit us on the starboard side amidships, just about the boundary between 2 and 3 boiler rooms, and at that, of course, the ship started to break up and it was a question of just getting out, and by the time I was able to get to the bridge, she was beginning to roll over on her beam ends, and LARRY RUTHERFORD and I were the last 2 on the bridge and we scrambled up and walked down the side of the ship and jumped into the sea.

GERMAN: Was the water very cold?

PULLEN: We were extremely fortunate — it's a good question — because we were just about on the boundary of the Canadian current and the Gulfstream. If the torpedoing had taken place just a few hours later we would have been in the cold water, and I suggest that probably very few would have survived. But as it was, the water temperature was bearable.

GERMAN: So did many remain in the water…?

PULLEN: Quite a few were lost in the water. An extraordinary thing to observe, men simply giving up and letting go the Carley

Floats, and drifting off into the night. I'm not quite sure why they would do this, because they were uninjured. I think probably shock and not being mentally geared to a catastrophe, after all, we were living in a catastrophic area at the time where a lot of ships were being sunk.

GERMAN: How many were lost, and how many survived?

PULLEN: We lost 113 officers and men, and about 65 survived, were picked up, and the survivors of the ship that we had picked up a few days earlier, we lost most of them in this torpedoing.

GERMAN: Tom, later you were involved in a successful anti-submarine action, could you just outline that?

PULLEN: Well after I'd completed my survivors leave, and I had spent some time at HMCS Cornwallis, I was agitated enough with Captain EDWARDS to get back to sea, and I was appointed to stand by and be 1st Lt. Of HMCS CHAUDIERE, and PAT NIXON was the Commanding Officer, and this was a very happy and efficient ship. We took her over in Plymouth, and became part of an escort group in the Atlantic, ET 11, and ST. CATHERINE's was the senior officer and we were working as a group in the Atlantic, West of Ireland, when a submarine contact was made by one of the ships, and this contact was hunted for a long time — day — hours — many, many hours, and it was a submarine and it eventually was forced to the surface and we discovered it was U-744 and she was surrounded by ships, and there was a certain amount of gunfire, they abandoned the submarine, she sank eventually, and we picked up some of the survivors.

GERMAN: Which ships were credited with the kill, Tom, do you remember?

PULLEN: Well I think the whole group was, because it was a group action, ST. CATHERINE's was the senior officer and I can't remember the names of the ships now...

GERMAN: Well Tom, perhaps you could contrast that sinking of OTTAWA with your later experience.

PULLEN: Yes, the loss of the OTTAWA of course, occurring in 1942, in the black days of the Battle of Atlantic, and it occurred, of course, in that area where air cover was not available, and radars weren't really all that good, but the tables began to turn, and in 1942 when I joined the CHAUDIERE as 1st Lt. — 1944 — I should say, the tide had turned in the Battle of the Atlantic, and the escorts were — had the situation I think pretty well in hand, and the submarines were rather on the defensive, and there was an incident in — in the — in which the escort group of which CHAUDIERE was a member, we located a submarine and hunted her to exhaustion and forced her to the surface — U-744, and this was a happy day for me because it sort of balanced the books a bit. CHAUDIERE, ICARUS, ST. CATHERINE's — and ST. CATHERINES was the senior officer, and the corvettes, CHILLIWACK and FENNELL, and the submarine was — once she surfaced, was scuttled and sank, and we picked up survivors, so that was a very successful outcome as far as we were concerned.

GERMAN: Was the submarine attacking the convoy, or were you a support group, or what was the situation?

PULLEN: No, the submarine was, I believe, located endeavouring to get in touch with the convoy, because we were acting as a support group of 5 ships, with a roving commission, which was meant that we could provide support to threatened convoys, and this in fact was what we were doing, and that's how we picked the submarine up.

GERMAN: Tom, you were Commanding Officer of Her Majesty's

Canadian Ship LABRADOR. Tell us about LABRADOR and your time in her.

PULLEN: Well HMCS LABRADOR was an icebreaker, and a very specialized ship, and at that time LABRADOR was the most modern and most marvellous ice-breaker that Canada had produced.

GERMAN: Could you tell us about your time in HMCS LABRADOR?

PULLEN: The happiest time in my Naval career, I had command of LABRADOR.

Notes

Prologue: A Burial at Sea

1   T.C. Pullen, "Convoy ON 127 & The Loss of HMCS *Ottawa*, 13 September 1942: A Personal Experience," *The Northern Mariner* II, no. 2 (April 1992): 1–27.

2   Pullen, "Convoy ON 127."

3   Latham B. Jenson, *Tin Hats, Oilskins and Seaboots: A Naval Journey 1938–45* (Toronto: Robin Brass Studio, 2000).

4   Pullen, "Convoy ON 127."

5   Ibid.

6   Jenson, *Tin Hats.*

7   "Then there was Bucheski [the recovering appendectomy patient] on whose behalf our gallant doctor, SBA MacMillan and Pooch's friends dedicated themselves to the task of saving him." Pullen, "Convoy ON 127," 15.

Chapter One: The Hendrys: A Remarkable Family

8   J.C. Goodwin, "William Belfry Hendry: An Appreciation," *Bulletin of the Academy of Medicine of Toronto* 12 (1939): 159.

9   "We all worship him." Michael Bliss, *William Osler: A Life in Medicine* (Toronto: University of Toronto Press, 1999), 208 ff.

10 On Sunday, March 31, 1929, George M. Hendry, a prominent businessman in Toronto, excused himself from the dinner table, walked out of his house at 104 Kilbarry Road, and disappeared. For the next several days, he was the subject of a citywide manhunt. Eight days later, he was found drowned in Grenadier Pond in west Toronto. An intensive investigation cleared any suspicion of foul play and an autopsy showed the cause of death to be asphyxia by drowning following an epileptic attack referred to at the time as "automatism."

11 In 1916, Colonel Hendry and his staff treated Lieutenant Robert Brown, the third officer of the famous British submarine E-11, for pneumonia. In gratitude, Brown gave Hendry a decommissioned battle

ensign from the submarine. In May and August 1915, E-11 had negotiated the very dangerous Dardanelles Straits and sunk a Turkish battleship and several other ships in the Sea of Marmora and Istanbul
Harbour. Her captain, Lieutenant Commander Martin Dunbar-
Nasmith, was awarded the Victoria Cross. After W.B. Hendry's death in
1939, his widow gave the ensign to my father, and it was in my family's
possession for many years. It now hangs in the "E-11 Room" of the
Royal Naval Submarine Museum in Gosport, Hampshire, U.K.

12   Resolution respecting the late William Belfry Hendry presented to
the Council of the Faculty of Medicine of the University of Toronto,
April 6, 1939.

13   J.W. Goodwin, "The Casebooks and Journals of a Toronto General
Hospital Houseman: J.C. Goodwin, MB, 1927–1928,"
J.Soc.Obstet.Gynec.Can. 23, no. 1 (2001): 45–52.

14   Resolution respecting the late Dr. James Clifford Goodwin presented to the Faculty of Medicine of the University of Medicine of the
University of Toronto, November 12, 1953.

15   Doctors smoked in those days: W.B. Hendry, George, my dad, and
many others. It wasn't till the emergence of all the damning evidence presented by the late Sir Richard Doll in the early 1960s on
the relationship between smoking and lung cancer that most
physicians stopped.

16   Three years after George died, Elizabeth Hendry sold the summer
house. The cottage was torn down and replaced by a small resort
called Bala Royal Lodge. Today, only the old boathouse remains.
See Bob Petry, *Bala: An Early Settlement in Muskoka* (Bracebridge,
ON: 1998), photograph and caption on page 196: "Bala Royal was
a small lodge and cottage resort on the Weismuller's Bay side of
Struan Point."

17   "As for Jews, institutional and social anti-semitism was for decades
the norm." Allan Levine, *The Devil in Babylon* (Toronto:
McClelland and Stewart, 2005), 38.

18   H.A. Bruce, "Sterilization of the Feeble-Minded," *Canadian
Medical Association Journal* 29 (1933): 260–263.

19   Calendar, Faculty of Medicine, University of Toronto, 1929–1930,
1934–1935.

20 Velma Demerson, *Incorrigible* (Waterloo, ON: Wilfrid Laurier University Press, 2004).

21 The Lord's Day Act (1907) restricted Sunday business "and fun." Allan Levine, *The Devil in Babylon: Fear of Progress and the Birth of Modern Life* (Toronto: McClelland and Stewart, 2005), 41.

22 Charis Cotter, *Toronto between the Wars: Life in the City 1919–1939* (Richmond Hill, ON: Firefly Books, 2004), 11.

Chapter Two: The Making of a Doctor: G.A. Hendry, Meds 3T5

23 Pierre Berton, *The Great Depression, 1929-1939* (Toronto: McClelland & Stewart, 1990).

24 Michiel Horn, *The Dirty Thirties: Canadians in the Great Depression* (Toronto: Copp Clark, 1972), 186.

25 Ibid., 535.

26 Piers Brendon and Phillip Whitehead, *The Windsors: A Dynasty Revealed* (London: BCA, 1994), opp. 142.

27 Horn, *The Dirty Thirties*, 194.

28 Ibid.

29 Christopher J. Rutty, "The Middle-Class Plague: Epidemic Polio and the Canadian State, 1936–1937," *Canadian Bulletin of Medical History* 13 (1996): 277–314.

30 Wendy Mitchinson, *Giving Birth in Canada, 1900–1950* (Toronto: University of Toronto Press, 2002).

31 Pierre Berton, *The Dionne Years: A Thirties Melodrama* (Toronto: McClelland & Stewart, 1977).

32 *The Toronto Daily Star*, Monday, July 13, 1936, p. 1 headline.

33 Horn, *The Dirty Thirties*, 204.

34 Calendar of the Faculty of Medicine, University of Toronto, 1934–35.

35 Given the expense of becoming a doctor in the 1930s, it is scarcely surprising that nearly one-third (29 percent) of medical students at the University of Toronto were the children of professionals and 39 percent were the sons and daughters of businessmen. (R.D. Gidney and W.P.J. Millar, "Medical Students at the University of Toronto, 1910–1940: A Profile," *Canadian Bulletin of Medical History* 13 [1996]: 29–52.)

36 J.C. Kwong et al, "Effects of Rising Tuition Fees on Medical School Class Composition and Financial Outlook," *Canadian Medical*

Association Journal 166, no. 8 (April 16, 2002): 1023–8.

37   Michael Bliss, *William Osler: A Life in Medicine* (Toronto: University of Toronto Press, 1999).

38   J.C.B. Grant, *A Method of Anatomy: Descriptive and Deductive*, 4th edition (Baltimore: The Williams and Wilkins Company, 1948).

39   C.L.N. Robinson, "J.C. Boileau Grant: Anatomist Extraordinary," in *Canadian Medical Lives*, ed. T.P. Morley (Toronto: AMS / Fitzhenry & Whiteside, 1993).

40   Ibid.

41   R.B. Kerr and D. Waugh, "Duncan Graham: Medical Reformer and Educator," in *Canadian Medical Lives*, ed. T.P. Morley (Toronto: Dundurn Press, 1989), 58–59.

42   C.T. Robertson (1911–98) told me this story when I was his assistant resident at Toronto East General Hospital in 1956. Feisty, tough, and very principled, he was a superb surgeon and a wonderful mentor who set high standards for himself and for others.

43   Ian Carr, "William Boyd. Silver Tongue and Golden Pen," in *Canadian Medical Lives*, ed. T.P. Morley (Toronto: AMS / Fitzhenry & Whiteside, 1993).

44   A.F. Kingsmill, "Dr. Alan Brown: Portrait of a Tyrant," *Canadian Medical Lives*, ed. T.P. Morley (Toronto: AMS / Fitzhenry & Whiteside, 1993).

45   J.C. Goodwin, "William Belfry Hendry: An appreciation," *Bulletin of the Academy of Medicine of Toronto* 21 (1939) 159.

46   Calendar for the Faculty of Medicine, University of Toronto, 1934–35.

47   J.T.H. Connor, *Doing Good: The Life of Toronto's General Hospital* (Toronto: The University of Toronto Press), 2002.

48   This venerable building was finally torn down to make way for the inevitable post-modern replacement on April 25, 2002, almost seventy-two years to the day after it was opened.

49   At the special convocation held in conjunction with this event, Professor W.B. Hendry will introduce Dr. Thomas S. Cullen ("Tom Cullen of Baltimore"), the distinguished professor of clinical gynecology at the Johns Hopkins Medical School and a graduate of Toronto Medical School for the degree of Doctor of Laws (LLD).

50 The inscription on the cane reads, "University of Toronto Medical Athletic Association. Presented to George A. Hendry, 1935. In Recognition of Athletic Honours."

51 When Colonel W.B. Hendry returned home after the Great War, he brought highland outfits for his sons, Jack and George, complete with kilt, sporran, jacket, and bonnet. When her boys had outgrown them, Mrs. Hendry gave these suits to our family for me and my younger brother John. When Their Majesties rode by in an open Landau carriage on their way out St. Clair Avenue West in Toronto to attend the Queen's Plate, there we were, turned out in our splendid highland livery, on the terraced lawn of the Hendry's home at 286 Russell Hill Road. We were just high enough above the cheering crowd on the sidewalk below that Queen Elizabeth (Scots to her marrow) could clearly see these two little boys in their Highland regalia and she waved at us! Our dear mother, always the unrepentant monarchist, never tired of relating this little imperial vignette.

52 Winston S. Churchill, *The Gathering Storm* (Boston: The Houghton Mifflin Company, 1948), 314–5.

Chapter Three: "Is Anxious to Have His Entry Hastened"

53 Queen Mary, in a letter to the Duke of Windsor, July 1938, published in James Pope-Hennessy, *Queen Mary, 1867–1953* (London: George Allen and Unwin, 1959), Chapter 7.

54 The Form of Registration of Marriage "sworn before me" (the Registrar) was made out in Toronto City Hall on March 29, 1941, five days before the marriage in Preston, Ontario, on April 3, 1941.

55 J.O. Cossette joined the primordial Royal Canadian Navy as a stoker in the venerable cruiser HMCS *Niobe* on its arrival in Halifax on October 21, 1910. Subsequently, he transferred to the ship's office as a writer or naval clerk and rose steadily through the ranks. He was commissioned and appointed naval secretary in 1940. Later, he became head of the Supply Branch and was the first rear-admiral (supply) in the RCN.

56 George's mother was driving with his aunt Mame from Toronto.

57 April 3, 1941, the date of the shotgun wedding in Preston, Ontario.

58 W.W. McLaughlin, 302 Bay Street, Toronto.

59 Dr. J. Fraser Macaulay graduated in medicine at McGill Medical School in 1896. One of Cape Breton's best known and most respected physicians, he practised in Sydney from 1916 until his death on July 3, 1943.

60 G.A. Hendry, "Obstetrical Difficulties," *Nova Scotia Medical Bulletin* 21 (March 1942): 124–129.

61 E.A. Minogue, communication with the author, January 14, 2003.

Chapter Four: HMCS *Ottawa* (H 60): The Ship and the Ship's Company

62 Nearly a year later, on October 14, 1942, SS *Caribou* was torpedoed and sunk by U-69 when on the same Sydney–Port Aux Basques run: 138 passengers and crew were lost, including 13 of the 14 children on board.

63 Jenson, *Tin Hats*.

64 As a lieutenant RNR in 1917, Cedric Naylor commanded the Q-ship *Penshurst* during several hair-raising battles with German submarines and was awarded the DSO with two bars and the DSC.

65 The details of this heroic encounter were not revealed until after the war's end. *Glowworm*'s captain, Lieutenant-Commander Gerard Broadmead Roope, RN, was lost just as he was being brought on board the *Hipper*. He was awarded the Victoria Cross posthumously on July 10, 1945.

66 Philip Zeigler, *Mountbatten: The Official Biography* (Glasgow: William Collins, 1985), 146.

67 During the war, there were hundreds of alphabetical codenames for convoys sailing to ports all over the world. For example:

TC: Canadian troop convoys, 1939–41 only.

OB: Liverpool outward bound, 1939–40 only.

HX: Halifax to United Kingdom (there were 358 of these between September 16, 1939, and May 23, 1945)

SC: Sydney, Nova Scotia, to United Kingdom

ON: Outward North United Kingdom to North America, initially to Halifax, then to New York.

PQ: Iceland to Russia.

68 Latham B. Jenson, "Events on 13 September 1942," a personal memoir to the author 2002.

69 Sid Dobing, letter to the author, December 6, 2002.

70 Jenson, *Tin Hats*, 122.

71 Elizabeth Pullen (T.C. Pullen's widow), letter to the author, March 1, 2002.

72 On January 26, 1985, in a taped interview with Commander Tony German, RCN (Ret'd), the author of *The Sea is at Our Gates: The History of the Canadian Navy*, Captain T.C. Pullen, RCN (Ret'd), described his life in the navy, the details of the surgery performed by Surgeon Lieutenant George Hendry (at which Pullen assisted), the sinking of HMCS *Ottawa*, and his postwar career as an outstanding Arctic navigator when he was commanding officer of the navy's great icebreaker, HMCS *Labrador*. It was in this interview that Tom Pullen looked back with such fondness to his time as a brand new sub-lieutenant in HMCS *Assiniboine* and with such affection for her captain, Commander (later Vice-Admiral) Rollo Mainguy, RCN. (See Appendix J.)

73 Jenson, *Tin Hats*, 126.

74 L.B. Jenson, letter to the author, May 18, 2002.

75 Ibid.

76 G. Beveridge, letter to the author, March 8, 2003.

77 Steve Logos, letter to the author, February 23, 2003.

78 Norm Wilson, letter to the author, December 23, 2006.

79 Pullen, "Convoy ON 127," 3.

Chapter Five: Into the Black Pit

80 Pullen, "Convoy ON 127," 3.

81 In a letter to Mrs. Walter Campbell dated August 12, 1981, Dr. Henry Swan wrote: "George Hendry and I were both born on Feb. 4, 1911 and sad to say was lost on the *Ottawa* just behind us. I had lunch with George in London just before that trip back to Canada."

82 W.R. Feasby, *Official History of the Canadian Medical Services 1939–1945 Volume I: Organization and Campaigns* (Ottawa: Department of National Defence, 1953), 121.

83 Pullen, "Convoy ON 127," 3. Pullen got the film into the post ashore before sailing. It was received at NSHQ on September 18.

84 David J. Bercuson and Holger H. Herwig, *Deadly Seas: The Duel*

Between the St. Croix *and the* U305 *in the Battle of the Atlantic* (Toronto: Random House Canada, 1997).

85 Ronald H. Spector, *At War At Sea: Sailors and Naval Combat in the Twentieth Century* (New York: Penguin Books, 2001), 232.

86 Chiefs of Staff Committee: Plan for the Defence of Canada, as amended to May 1939. PAC, RG 24, 2696, HQS 5199, F, V I.

87 Jenson, *Tin Hats*, 33.

88 German, *The Sea*, 68.

89 Ibid.

90 David Zimmerman, *The Great Naval Battle of Ottawa* (Toronto: University of Toronto Press, 1989), 17–18.

91 W.A.B. Douglas, Roger Sarty, and Michael Whitby, *No Higher Purpose: The Official Operational History of the Royal Canadian Navy, Vol. II, Part I: 1939–1943* (Ottawa and St. Catharines, ON: Vanwell Publishing and Department of National Defence, 2003), 305–306.

92 Zimmerman, *The Great Naval Battle*, 24–25.

93 Marc Milner, *North Atlantic Run: The Royal Canadian Navy and the Battle for the Convoys* (Toronto: University of Toronto Press, 1985), 77.

94 Zimmerman, *The Great Naval Battle*, 72–73.

95 Douglas, Sarty, and Whitby, *No Higher Purpose*, 115.

96 Ibid., 305–6.

97 Milner, *North Atlantic Run*, 140.

98 Zimmerman, *The Great Naval Battle*, 78.

99 Latham B. Jenson to W.A.B. Douglas, cited in Pullen, "Convoy ON 127," 24.

100 Douglas, Sarty, and Whitby, *No Higher Purpose*, foldout map opposite p. 488.

101 Excerpt from an interview of Bob Bromley, a veteran Merchant Navy sailor, conducted by Norman Date (Hon. Secretary, Merchant Navy Association, Britol, U.K.) as part of a BBC archival presentation entitled *WW2 People's War*, November 1, 2003 (reproduced with permission of Norman Date):

> I joined the tanker *Empire Oil* on the 10th August 1942. We sailed from Avonmouth on about the 20th August 1942 and at Swansea loaded with petrol bound for Malta

or Russia. Our orders were changed and we discharged the cargo and sailed with water ballast from Milford Haven to Belfast from where on the 5th September 1942 we joined convoy ON-127 for our journey across the North Atlantic. On the 10th September we were torpedoed in the engine-room, killing two crewmen and injuring gunlayer Jones, who was coming out of his cabin when a rivet driven from the plates by the explosion, hit him in the stomach. Gunlayer Jones* subsequently died from this injury and was buried at sea from HMCS *Ottawa* prior to her being torpedoed.

*Jones, Able Seaman Thomas Brynmor P/JX289340 HMS *President III* Royal Navy. (Lost in *Empire Oil* 13 September 1942) Age 22. Husband of Mary Elizabeth Jones, Redditch, Worcestershire.

Chapter Six: "Doctor in His Cabin Operating Room Hero of Plunging *Ottawa*"

102 Headline for article in *Toronto Daily Star*, September 26, 1942.

103 Pullen, "Convoy ON 127," 6.

104 W.C. MacKenzie, "Surgical Problems in the Royal Canadian Navy," *Canadian Medical Association Journal* 47 (1942): 443–7.

105 Surgeon Lieutenant-Commander C.M. Oake, RCNVR, "Medical Organization in Destroyers," DHH 4430 Medical Branch (Pamphlets and Pharmacy) 1943.

106 Pullen, "Convoy ON 127," 6.

107 S.T. Richards, *Operation Sick Bay: The Story of the Sick Berth and Medical Assistant Branch of the Royal Canadian Navy, 1910–1965* (West Vancouver: Cantaur Publishing, 1994). This book has a diagram of the ship's layout that shows just how small the sick bay actually was.

108 Oake, "Medical Organization in Destroyers," 18.

109 Admiralty Fleet Orders (AFO) #2530 "Scale of Medicines and Instruments" (dated 4.7.40).

110 Pullen, "Convoy ON 127," 6.

111 Richards, *Operation Sick Bay*.

112 Dr. Bruce A. Campbell graduated in medicine at the University of Western Ontario in 1939, interned at the Hamilton General Hospital, and joined the RCNVR in December 1940. Subsequently, he served as medical officer on the destroyer HMCS *Assiniboine* for eleven months before being posted to the Royal Navy and to the ship in which he performed this surgery. After the war, Bruce Campbell did postgraduate training in London, Ontario, and practised general surgery for the next thirty years in Stratford and New Liskeard. He died on July 26, 1993, in Tiverton, Ontario.

113 Press Release, Medical Branch, Vol. 2 DHH 4430.

114 Jan K. Herman, *Battle Station Sick Bay: Navy Medicine in World War II* (Annapolis, MD: The Naval Institute Press, 1997), 119–28.

115 Pullen, "Convoy ON 127," 8–10.

116 Pullen, "Convoy ON 127," 9.

117 Rodney Maingot, "Injuries of the Intestines," in *Abdominal Operations, Volume II* (New York: Appleton-Century, 1940).

118 R. Maingot, E.G. Slesinger, and E. Fletcher, *War Wounds and Injuries* (London: Edward Arnold & Co., 1940).

119 "Doctor in His Cabin Operating-Room, Hero of Plunging *Ottawa*," *Toronto Daily Star*, September 26, 1942.

120 Pullen, "Convoy ON 127," 10.

121 In his textbook on war wounds and injuries, Rodney Maingot set down the following advice:

In examining the hollow viscera (like the intestine) for abdominal injury, it is wise to proceed on a definite plan.... The following rules should be borne in mind in the inspection of intestinal wounds:

1. The small intestine is the part damaged in the great majority of these cases and this portion must be inspected loop by loop, starting at the ileocaecal junction (the junction of the small and large bowel in right lower corner of the abdominal cavity) and proceeding upwards.

2. Inspect the small intestine once and once only; make up your mind at the first examination. There must be no

re-examination.

3. Withdraw each loop in an orderly fashion, and then replace it in the abdomen. The patient is already shocked; rough handling will augment shock and jeopardise his life.

4. Remember the possibility of wounds between the layers of the mesenteric attachment.

5. A single layer of suture suffices for the repair of the small bowel.

6. Escape of bowel contents (with its E.Coli bacterial contamination) takes place more quickly after wounds of the colon (large bowel) than in the small gut (intestine). The prognosis may thus rapidly become hopeless.

7. Remember the importance of adequate drainage in retroperitoneal colonic injuries and the local use of sulphanilamide.

8. Drain the retroperitoneal tissues lavishly whenever they are contaminated. (large bowel injuries could leak faeces into the tisses behind the peritoneum, causing lethal E.Coli infection).

9. If after dealing with a tear in the mesentery, an adjacent portion of bowel takes on a mauve tint, or becomes dark brown in colour, it is best to assume that the involved segment is lifeless, (this would require its resection and re-anastamosis or joining together of the healthy small bowel).

122 Pullen, "Convoy ON 127," 9–10.

123 Pullen, "Convoy ON 127," 9–10.

124 W.G.P. Rawling, *Death Their Enemy: Canadian Medical Practitioners and War* (Ottawa: privately published, 2001).

125 Pullen, "Convoy ON 127."

126 Ibid.

Chapter Seven: "She Was a Fine Ship, Number One"

127 Zulu = Greenwich Mean Time.

128 A twenty-four-hour day is divided into watches. The "first watch" is from 2000 (8:00 p.m.) to 2400 (midnight), the "middle watch"

from 2400 to 0400 (4:00 a.m.), the "morning watch" from 0400 to 0800 (8:00 a.m.), the "forenoon watch" from 0800 to 1200 (noon), the "afternoon watch" from 1200 to 1600 (4:00 p.m.), the "first dog watch" from 1600 to 1800 (6:00 p.m.) and the "second dog watch" from 1800 to 2000.

129   "Our Gunner(T) (for Torpedo Gunner) was Mr. Lloyd Jones, promoted from the ranks and given a Warrant, a type of commission with the full status of a commissioned officer. Many of these gentlemen were later promoted to Lieutenant and higher; some even made Admiral! I have to say that I really admired Lloyd Jones, an 'old man' of 32 versus my 21 years. What a fine, wise, experienced gentleman he was!" Latham B. Jenson, unpublished memoirs of September 13, 1942.

130   Latham B. Jenson, "Sinking of HMCS *Ottawa*," in Ian Maxwell, ed. *This Was My War: A Collection of Twelve Essays on the 1939–1945 Conflict* (Tancook Island, NS: Little Daisy Press, 1992).

131   *Toronto Daily Star*, September 26, 1942: "Doctor in his cabin operating-room hero of plunging *Ottawa*."

132   Jenson, "Sinking of HMCS *Ottawa*." in Ian Maxwell, ed. *This Was My War: A Collection of Twelve Essays on the 1939–1945 Conflict* (Tancook Island, NS: Little Daisy Press, 1992).

133   Jenson, *Tin Hats.*

134   Jenson, *Tin Hats.*

135   C.R. Skillen, letter to the author, February 2, 2003.

136   "Hydrophone effect" is a sonic phenomenon caused by the noise generated by the screws (propellers) of approaching ships. Pullen, "Convoy ON 127," 12.

137   Pullen, "Convoy ON 127," 12.

138   "Grain" is a seaman's term for the line of water ahead of a vessel along which she will pass. The opposite of wake. Admiralty Manual of Seamanship Vol II, London 1952, 746.

139   Pullen, "Convoy ON 127," 1–27.

140   Oblt z. S. Heinz Walkerling in U-91's KTB (*Kriegstagebuch*, or War Diary). (See Appendix I.)

141   Pullen, "Convoy ON 127," 1–27.

142   *Schussmeldung* (torpedo shot report) of U-91. (See Appendix I.)

143   Walkerling in U-91's KTB.

144 The two forward guns on a warship are labelled "A" and "B", "A" being nearest the bow. The rear guns are "X" and "Y", "Y" gun being next to the stern. In 1942, *Ottawa*'s "Y" gun was removed to make increased freedom of action for the depth charge crews.

145 Latham B. Jenson, "Sinking of HMCS *Ottawa*," in Ian Maxwell, ed. *This Was My War: A Collection of Twelve Essays on the 1939–1945 Conflict* (Tancook Island, NS: Little Daisy Press, 1992).

146 Pullen, "Convoy ON 127," 1–27.

147 Steve Logos, letter to the author, February 23, 2003.

148 Sid Dobing, letter to the author, December 6, 2002.

149 Al Underhill, letter to the author, March 6, 2003.

150 Jenson, *Tin Hats*.

151 Bercuson and Herwig, *Deadly Seas*, 219–20.

152 ROP (Report of Proceedings) for *St. Croix*, SOE Task Unit 24.1.14, escorting Convoy ON 127. (See Appendix G.)

153 ROP for HMS *Witch*. (See Appendix H.)

154 *Schussmeldung* (torpedo shot report) of U-91. (See Appendix I.)

155 Excerpt from War Diary for U-91. (See Appendix I.)

156 ROP for *St. Croix*. (See Appendix G.)

157 ROP for HMS *Witch*. (See Appendix H.)

158 Bercuson and Herwig, *Deadly Seas*, 219–20.

159 ROP for *St. Croix*. (See Appendix G.)

160 Latham B. Jenson, "Sinking of HMCS *Ottawa*," in Ian Maxwell, ed. *This Was My War: A Collection of Twelve Essays on the 1939–1945 Conflict* (Tancook Island, NS: Little Daisy Press, 1992).

161 Pullen, "Convoy ON 127," 1–27.

162 Ibid.

163 Al Underhill, letter to the author, March 6, 2003.

164 *Toronto Daily Star*. September 26, 1942: "Doctor in his cabin operating room hero of plunging Ottawa."

165 A Carley float was rather like a large oblong rubber doughnut, roughly twelve feet long by seven feet wide. Linked rope lanyards were tightly strapped around the rim of the float at intervals of two feet. These lanyards were so tightly applied that it was difficult even for well-rested men to cling to a float in calm seas. But at night in a rising sea, it was virtually impossible for exhausted men to hold them.

166 *Toronto Daily Star.* September 26, 1942: "Doctor in his cabin operating room hero of plunging Ottawa."

167 C. Roe Skillen, letter to the author, February 2, 2003.

168 George D. Johnson, letter to the author, July 18, 2003.

169 Pullen, "Convoy ON 127," 1–27.

170 Pullen, "Convoy ON 127," 15–16.

171 Ibid.

172 Norm Wilson, letter to the author, December 23, 2006.

173 Sid Dobing, letter to the author, December 6, 2002.

174 The legendary "Mae West" was so named because when tied around the chest, this apparatus seemed to simulate a voluptuous bosom, for which Ms. West was justifiably famous.

175 Latham B. Jenson, "Sinking of HMCS *Ottawa*," in Ian Maxwell, ed. *This Was My War: A Collection of Twelve Essays on the 1939–1945 Conflict* (Tancook Island, NS: Little Daisy Press, 1992).

176 Ibid.

177 Al Underhill, letter to the author, March 6, 2003.

178 C.R. Skillen, letter to the author, February 2, 2003.

179 Sid Dobing, letter to the author, December 6, 2002.

180 Steve Logos, letter to the author, February 23, 2002.

181 Pullen, "Convoy ON 127," 1–27.

182 Norm Wilson, letter to the author, December 23, 2006.

183 Ibid.

184 On September 22, 1914, in an area of the North Sea off the Dutch coast called the "Broad Fourteens," the old armoured cruiser HMS *Aboukir* was torpedoed by the German submarine U-9 (Kapitän-Leutnant Otto Weddigen). A second old cruiser, HMS *Hogue*, went to the aid of her stricken sister and she was torpedoed. A third cruiser, HMS *Cressy*, hurried in to rescue the crews of the other two and she too was dispatched by U-9. The loss of life was enormous: 1,400 seamen drowned, including many thirteen- and fourteen-year-old cadet midshipmen. The pictures of these boys in the pages of the *Illustrated London News* reporting the disaster are truly haunting. From that day, there seems to have been an unwritten order from the Admiralty that warships (or indeed any ship) were forbidden to go to the aid of a torpedoed sister ship.

185 Years later, Jenson "asked this gentleman who was by now a Lieutenant, why he had been so kind and good to me. When I was on the famous 'Newfie Bullet' [the train to St. John's] traveling to join *Ottawa*, his wife and a shipmate's wife were going to St. John's to be closer to their husbands. Evidently, I had taken them to dinner and been pleasant and helpful to them. I had no recollection of this other than just meeting two nice ladies, but my reward had been great." (Jenson, *Tin Hats*, 140.)

186 Pullen, "Convoy ON 127," 19.

187 Sid Dobing, letter to the author, December 6, 2002.

188 C.R. Skillen, letter to the author, February 2, 2003.

189 Sid Dobing, letter to the author, Decmeber 6, 2002.

190 Steve Logos, letter to the author, February 23, 2003.

191 Norm Wilson, letter to the author, December 23, 2006.

192 "The Ties That Bind," *The Humber Log*, November 5, 1997.

193 Jenson, *Tin Hats*.

Chapter Eight: "The Most Commendable Devotion to Duty"

194 See Appendix F for complete list of *Ottawa's* survivors.

195 Jenson, *Tin Hats*.

196 Steve Logos, letter to the author, February 23, 2003.

197 See Appendix E for *Ottawa's* casualty list.

198 Steve Logos, letter to the author, February 23, 2003.

199 Jenson, *Tin Hats*.

200 Milner, *North Atlantic Run*.

201 Ibid.

202 Ibid.

203 Improbably, *zaunkönig* is the German for "wren."

204 Bercuson and Herwig, *Deadly Seas*, 263–75; Fraser McKee and Robert Darlington, *The Canadian Naval Chronicle, 1939–1945: The Successes and Losses of the Canadian Navy in World War II* (St. Catharines, ON: Vanwell Publishing, 1996), 102–105; and Marc Milner, *The U-Boat Hunters: The Royal Canadian Navy and the Offensive against Germany's Submarines* (Toronto: University of Toronto Press, 1994), 67–70.

205 The only decorations awarded posthumously to British and Commonwealth servicemen during the Second World War were the

Victoria Cross and the Mention in Despatches.

206 Sid Dobing, letter to the author, December 6, 2002.

Epilogue: A Closed Book

207 The following paean, "The Long Shadows," written in rather ornate language, was published as the last paragraphs in an article on ethical conduct (J.B. McClinton, "The Doctor's Own Ethics," *Canadian Medical Association Journal* 52 [1945]: 202) as an apparent tribute to the late Dr. W.B. Hendry and his sons, the late Dr. W.J. (Jack) Hendry and the late Dr. George A. Hendry:

THE LONG SHADOWS

The dinner was well appointed and it was at seven. Restless beams from the candelabra played hide and seek through the rose goblets. They danced off English silver. They brushed the Spode tureen.

The guest was quite at home. He lifted his soup as nonchalantly as he wore scholastic laurels years before. He never told that he could wear the Professor's gown at the Faculty. Nor that he carried the gold headed cane for the best athlete. His high rank in the World War I was just routine.

He left his knife parallel to his fork. His spoon lay beside his cup. He addressed a clinical meeting in a most scholarly manner. That was fifteen years before his last coronary.

He must have bequeathed something, for his two sons were like him. One a research fellow reached his white sleeved arm too far and the animal bit him. Polio viruses are small, not understood and virulent. The boy was so young to be so still and white.

The other was ship's surgeon. The torpedo left only the stern. He stayed till all were off. He gave morphine and left some crimson drops along the deck. The stern dipped down and the water met him cold. He swam to a

raft and reached one arm up … but let go. He turned
once more and grasped the cable … a depth charge
hurled him away. He worked slowly back and climbed
again but the raft tipped. Seven times in all he tried and
then a large grey sea closed over.

And now the silvery shoals of porpoise leap and
winged gulls descend, and flimsy tufts of mist float down
to kiss the grey green waves. Or sometimes skipping
whirlwinds push the sea and whitecaps break. While far
below he sleeps and far above a finger moves … to write
his name in immortality.

208   From a transcript of an interview of Captain T.C. Pullen, RCN
(Ret'd), by Commander Tony German, RCN (Ret'd), on January 26,
1985: in answer to a question about Tom Pullen's command of
Labrador, 1956–57.

209   Rowley, Graham, "Captain T.C. Pullen, RCN: Polar Navigator,"
The Northern Mariner II, no. 2 (April 1992): 29–49.

210   Ibid.

211   C.R. Skillen, letter to the author, February 2, 2003.

212   Al Underhill, letter to the author, March 6, 2003.

213   Sid Dobing, letter to the author, December 6, 2003.

214   Steve Logos, letter to the author, February 23, 2003.

215   "The Ties That Bind," *The Humber Log*, November 5, 1997.

216   Nancy Blanchette (Terry Terrabassi's daughter), letter to the author,
May 12, 2005.

217   Susan Minogue, letter to the author, May 29, 2006.

218   Craig Somerville's grandfather was Robert Charles Matthews, the
minister of national revenue in R.B. Bennett's cabinet in 1933 and
brother to Alfred Joseph Matthews, Jean's father, who was killed in
action in Flanders in February 1916. Thus, Jean and Craig were
indeed second cousins.

219   Fred E. Bryans is professor and chairman emeritus of obstetrics and
gynaecology of the University of British Columbia.

Bibliography

Bercuson, David J., and Holger H. Herwig. *Deadly Seas: The Duel Between the* St. Croix *and the* U305 *in the Battle of the Atlantic*. Toronto: Random House Canada, 1997.

Berton, Pierre. *Marching as to War: Canada's Turbulent Years, 1899–1953*. Toronto: Doubleday Canada, 2001.

———. *The Great Depression 1929-1939*. Toronto: McClelland & Stewart, 1990.

———. *The Joy of Writing: A Guide for Writers Disguised as a Literary Memoir*. Toronto: Doubleday Canada, 2003.

———. *Worth Repeating: A Literary Resurrection*. Toronto: Doubleday Canada, 1998.

Bliss, Michael. *Banting: A Biography*. Toronto: McClelland & Stewart, 1984.

———. *William Osler: A Life in Medicine*. Toronto: University of Toronto Press, 2001.

Carr, Ian. "William Boyd: Silver Tongue and Golden Pen." In *Canadian Medical Lives*, edited by T.P. Morley. Toronto: AMS / Fitzhenry & Whiteside, 1993.

Chatterton, E. Keble. *Q-Ships and Their Story*. London: Sidgwick and Jackson, 1923.

Cotter, Charis. *Toronto between the Wars: Life in the City 1919–1939*. Richmond Hill: Firefly Books Inc., 2004.

Douglas, W.A.B., Roger Sarty, and Michael Whitby. *No Higher Purpose: The Official Operational History of the Royal Canadian Navy in the Second World War*, Volume II Part I. Ottawa and St. Catharines, ON: Vanwell Publishing and Department of National Defence, 2003.

Feasby, W.R. *Official History of the Canadian Medical Services 1939–1945. Volume I: Organization and Campaigns. Volume II: Clinical Subjects*. Ottawa: Department of National Defence, 1953.

Filey, Mike. *Toronto Sketches: "The Way We Were"*. Toronto: Dundurn Press, 1992.

German, Tony. *The Sea is at Our Gates.* Toronto: McClelland & Stewart, 1990.

Goodwin, J.W. "The Casebooks and Journals of a Toronto General Hospital Houseman: J.C. Goodwin, MB, 1927–1928." *J. Soc. Obstet. Gynaecol. Can.* 23, no. 1 (2001): 45–52.

Graves, Donald E. *In Peril on the Sea. The Royal Canadian Navy and the Battle of the Atlantic.* Toronto: Robin Brass Studio, 2003.

Greenfield, Nathan M. *The Battle of the St. Lawrence.* Toronto: HarperCollins, 2004.

Hague, Arnold. *The Allied Convoy System 1939–1945: Its Organization, Defence and Operation.* Annapolis, MD: The Naval Institute Press, 2000.

Harbron, John D. *The Longest Battle: The Royal Canadian Navy in the Atlantic, 1939–1945.* St. Catharines, ON: Vanwell Publishing, 1995.

Herman, Jan K. *Battle Station Sick Bay: Navy Medicine in World War II.* Annapolis, MD: The Naval Institute Press, 1997.

Jane, F.T. Jane's Fighting Ships, 1939. *London: Sampson Low Marston, 1939.*

Jenson, Latham B. *Tin Hats, Oilskins and Seaboots: A Naval Journey 1938–45.* Toronto: Robin Brass Studio, 2000.

Keegan, John. *The Price of Admiralty: The Evolution of Naval Warfare.* London: Century Hutchinson Ltd., 1988.

Kerr, R.B., and D. Waugh. "Duncan Graham: Medical Reformer and Educator." In *Canadian Medical Lives*, edited by T.P. Morley. Toronto: Dundurn Press, 1989.

Kimber, Stephen. *Sailors, Slackers and Blind Pigs: Halifax at War.* Toronto: Doubleday Canada, 2002.

Kingsmill, A.F. "Dr. Alan Brown: Portrait of a Tyrant." In *Canadian Medical Lives*, edited by T.P. Morley. Toronto: AMS / Fitzhenry & Whiteside, 1993.

Lamb, James B. *The Corvette Navy: True Stories from Canada's Atlantic War,* 2nd Edition. Toronto: Stoddart, 2000.

Lynch, Thomas G., ed. *Fading Memories: Canadian Sailors and the Battle of the Atlantic.* Halifax, NS: The Atlantic Chief and Petty Officers Association, 1993.

MacPherson, Ken. *River Class Destroyers of the Royal Canadian Navy.* Toronto: C.J. Musson, 1985.

Macpherson, Ken, and Marc Milner. *Corvettes of the Royal Canadian Navy 1939–1945*. St. Catharines, ON: Vanwell Publishing, 2000.

Macpherson, Ken, and Ron Barrie. *The Ships of Canada's Naval Forces 1910–2002*. St. Catharines, ON: Vanwell Publishing, 2002.

Maingot, Rodney. "Injuries of the Intestines." In *Abdominal Operations, Volume II*. New York: Appleton-Century, 1940.

Maingot, Rodney, E.G. Slesinger, and Ernest Fletcher, eds. *War Wounds and Injuries*. London: Edward Arnold & Co., 1940.

McKee, Fraser M., and Robert A. Darlington. *The Canadian Naval Chronicle, 1935–45: The Successes and Losses of the Canadian Navy in World War II*. St. Catharines, ON: Vanwell Publishing, 1996.

Milner, Marc. *Battle of the Atlantic*. St. Catharines, ON: Vanwell Publishing, 2003.

———. *North Atlantic Run: The Royal Canadian Navy and the Battle for the Convoys*. Toronto: University of Toronto Press, 1985.

———. *The U-Boat Hunters: The Royal Canadian Navy and the Offensive Against Germany's Submarines*. Toronto: University of Toronto Press, 1994.

———. *Canada's Navy: The First Century*. Toronto: University of Toronto Press, 1999.

Mitchinson, Wendy. *Giving Birth in Canada, 1900–1950*. Toronto: University of Toronto Press, 2002.

Pullen, T.C. "Convoy ON 127 & The Loss of HMCS *Ottawa*, 13 September 1942: A Personal Experience." *The Northern Mariner* II, no. 2 (April 1992): 1–27.

Rawling, Bill. "Taking Care of Tar: The Royal Canadian Navy Medial Practitioners of the Second World War." *War & Society* 16, no. 2 (1998): 59–70.

———. *Death Their Enemy: Canadian Medical Practitioners and War*. Ottawa: privately published, 2001.

Robinson, C.L.N. "J.C. Boileau Grant: Anatomist Extraordinary." In *Canadian Medical Lives*, edited by T.P. Morley. Toronto: AMS / Fitzhenry & Whiteside, 1993.

Sarty, Roger. *Canada and the Battle of the Atlantic*. Montreal: Art Global and the Department of National Defence, 1998.

Schull, Joseph. *The Far Distant Ships: An Official Account of Canadian*

Naval Operations in the Second World War. Toronto: Stoddart, 1987.

Spector, Ronald H. *At War At Sea: Sailors and Naval Combat in the Twentieth Century.* New York: Penguin Books, 2001.

Tuchman, Barbara. *Practicing History: Selected Essays.* New York: Alfred A. Knopf, 1981.

White, Randall. *Too Good to be True: Toronto in the 1920s.* Toronto: Dundurn Press, 1993.

Zimmerman, David. *The Great Naval Battle of Ottawa.* Toronto: University of Toronto Press, 1989.

Index